Neuropathology Simplified

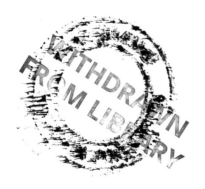

David A. Hilton • Aditya G. Shivane

Neuropathology Simplified

A Guide for Clinicians and Neuroscientists

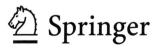
Springer

David A. Hilton
Cellular and Anatomical Pathology Level 4
Derriford Hospital
Plymouth
UK

Aditya G. Shivane
Cellular and Anatomical Pathology Level 4
Derriford Hospital
Plymouth
UK

ISBN 978-3-319-14604-1   ISBN 978-3-319-14605-8   (eBook)
DOI 10.1007/978-3-319-14605-8

Library of Congress Control Number: 2015933633

Springer Cham Heidelberg New York Dordrecht London

Printed on acid-free paper

Springer is part of Springer Science+Business Media (www.springer.com)

For Angela who has put up with my repeated absences whilst working on the book.
David A. Hilton

I dedicate this book to my parents.
To Veena, Diya and Neel for their patience and endless support.
Aditya G. Shivane

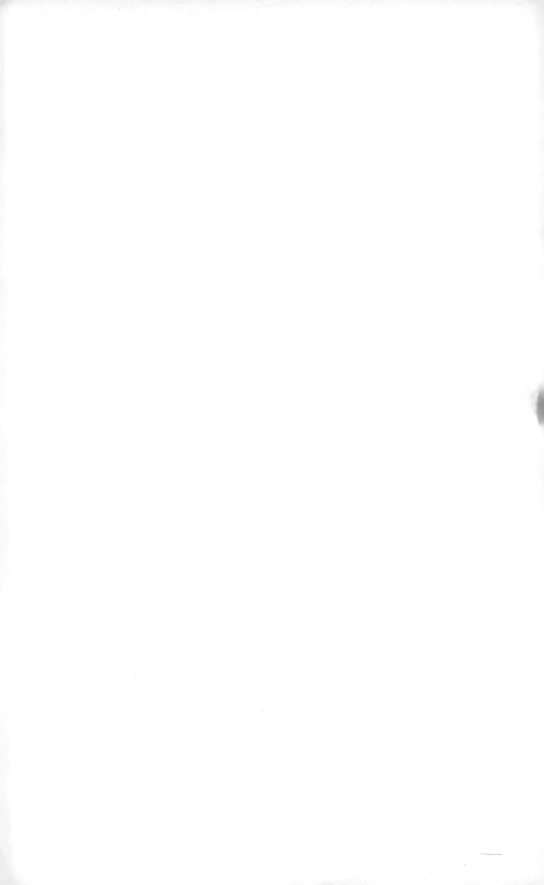

Preface

Neuropathology is a highly specialised branch of histopathology or anatomical pathology which deals with the gross and microscopic examination of tissues of the nervous system thereby aiding the clinicians in the diagnosis of disease. A neuropathologist also examines skeletal muscle and peripheral nerve tissue removed as a part of evaluation in patients with neuromuscular conditions.

The field of neuropathology is quite vast and has witnessed immense growth in the last decade with ever increasing research and rapid translation of basic science into clinical practice. It is not possible for a trainee or resident in clinical specialities like neurology, neurosurgery or psychiatry to receive all the training in neuropathology during their curricula nor can they keep up with the rapid advances in the scientific techniques and concepts. With the introduction of multi-disciplinary team approach, there is much need for clinical residents or trainees to have a sound knowledge of basic neuropathology in order to better understand and keep pace with the recent advances in neurological disorders.

This book will aim to provide the reader with an up-to-date, practical and succinct overview of basic neuropathology. This book will certainly not replace the existing large reference textbooks in neuropathology, but will rather emphasize key concepts and basic principles including recent advances, genetics, and classification, discuss important aspects of specific neuropathological disorders and also give practical hints on some aspects of neuropathology, including how to best use the neuropathology service and interpret the results of pathological tests.

The book is organised into 15 chapters and follows a standard text disease groupings. The chapters are quick and easy to read, focussing on practically relevant information. We have tried to richly illustrate the book where possible with diagrams and charts, thereby assisting the reader in recognising the morphology of various neuropathological conditions. The book also emphasises the clinico-pathologic correlations where necessary.

We sincerely hope that the readers of this book will achieve a sufficiently broad basic knowledge of neuropathology which will eventually help in their future clinical careers.

Finally, we would like to thank Ms. Joanna Ford and Mr. Philip Edwards for their excellent assistance in the preparation of the manuscript. Our thanks to Ms. Joanna Bolesworth and the team at Springer for giving us an opportunity to write this book.

Plymouth, UK   David A. Hilton
Plymouth, UK   Aditya G. Shivane

Contents

Chapter 1
Normal Histology and Commonly Used Stains

Abstract An understanding of the pathology of human nervous system requires a good basic knowledge of the normal cellular components and their architecture. This chapter starts with the discussion of normal cellular constituents of the nervous system, their morphology and some of their salient functions. The general architecture of central and peripheral nervous tissues is then described. The nervous tissue and their various components are studied using traditional tinctorial stains. Immunohistochemical preparations which target specific cellular antigens are now being increasingly used for both diagnostic and research purposes.

Keywords Cells • Histology • Nervous system • Stains • Immunohistochemistry

The human nervous system can be broadly divided into two parts- the central and peripheral nervous system. The central nervous system (CNS) includes the brain and spinal cord. Both brain and spinal cord are surrounded by tough coverings called the meninges and are encased in a protective bony structure, the skull and the vertebral column respectively. The peripheral nervous system (PNS) includes the nerves (cranial, spinal and peripheral nerves), sensory ganglia (dorsal root ganglion) and autonomic ganglia (sympathetic and parasympathetic ganglia).

1.1 Cells of the Nervous System

The cells which make up the nervous system are the neurons and other supporting cells (glial cells) which include astrocytes, oligodendrocytes, Schwann cells, ependymal cells and microglia.

1.1.1 Neurons

A neuron is the basic functional unit of the nervous system. It is primarily responsible for collecting information, processing and then generating response. During development, they are derived from the neural tube and eventually migrate and

© Springer International Publishing Switzerland 2015
D.A. Hilton, A.G. Shivane, *Neuropathology Simplified: A Guide for Clinicians and Neuroscientists*, DOI 10.1007/978-3-319-14605-8_1

populate different regions of the nervous system. A neuron is a post-mitotic cell and therefore cannot be replaced when damaged. It is also a highly metabolically active cell and requires continuous supply of nutrition for normal functioning. In an adult brain, neural stem cells have been identified within the subventricular zone of lateral ventricles, in the dentate gyrus of hippocampus and in the olfactory bulb.

The basic structure of a neuron include a cell body or *perikaryon*, many short processes or dendrites which receive information from other neurons and a single long process called 'axon' which transmits signals to other neurons. The dendrites and axons are collectively referred to as neurites. The cell body appears large in some types of neurons and contains a large nucleus with a prominent nucleolus. The cytoplasm of the neuron also contain granular dark staining material rich in rough endoplasmic reticulum termed *'Nissl substance'* which is one of the important distinguishing feature on microscopy (Figs. 1.1a and 1.2; Box 1.1). The region where axon begins is called an 'axon hillock' from where action potentials are generated.

The neurons come in various shapes and sizes. Neurons in some locations such as dentate gyrus and cerebellum appear small and rounded with no visible cytoplasm and are referred to as granular neurons. Neurons can be either multipolar (many dendrites, single axon. e.g. motor neurons), bipolar (single dendrite, single axon. e.g. sensory neurons in retina) or unipolar/pseudo-unipolar (single process which divides into central and peripheral axons, no dendrites. e.g. sensory neurons in dorsal root ganglia). The majority of neurons within the nervous system are multipolar (Fig. 1.1b).

The cell bodies of neurons make up the bulk of grey matter and deep nuclei of the brain and spinal cord. Their axons run as bundles within the white matter. Occasional neurons can be seen within the white matter, especially in the temporal lobe. This should not be mistaken for a neuronal migration abnormality.

Box 1.1 How to Identify a Neuron
Large cell and cell body
Large nucleus
Single prominent nucleolus
Nissl substance (purplish granules on H&E)

1.1.2 Astrocytes

Astrocytes are the most numerous of the glial cells and give structural and metabolic support to a neuron. Astrocytes are derived from radial glial cells during embryonic development. Astrocytes appear to have several complex roles in healthy tissue, some of which include- development of grey and white matter, regulation of blood flow, maintaining biochemical homeostasis, synapse function, and CNS

Fig. 1.1 (**a**) Diagram showing different parts of a neuron and, (**b**) the basic morphological subtypes of neurons

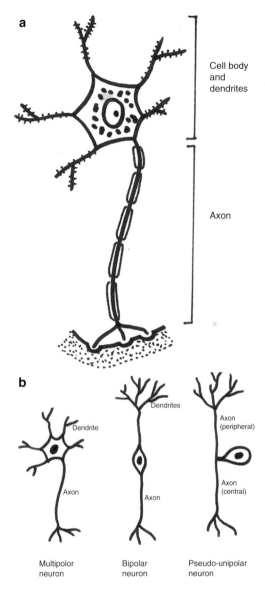

metabolism [1]. Astrocytes have star-shaped cytoplasmic processes which can be identified with a special stain such as phosphotungstic acid haematoxylin (PTAH) (Fig. 1.3 and Box 1.2). These processes abut on capillaries, neuron, axon, dendrites and pia mater (the innermost layer of meninges). The cytoplasmic processes contain characteristic filaments termed 'glial fibrillary acidic protein' or GFAP which can be demonstrated using immunohistochemistry. Astrocytes can be of two

Fig. 1.2 A cortical
pyramidal neuron showing a
large nucleus, prominent
nucleolus and purplish
granules (Nissl substance)
in the cytoplasm (*arrow*).
H&E stain

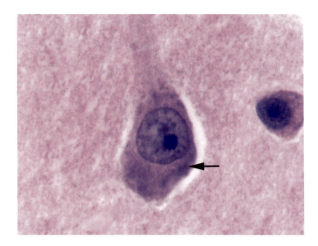

Fig. 1.3 Fibrous or fibrillary
astrocytes with stellate
cytoplasmic processes
(*arrows*). PTAH stain

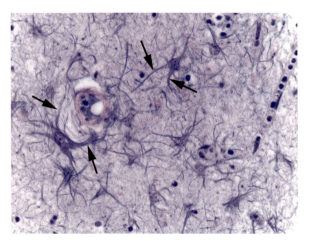

morphological subtypes- (1) fibrous or fibrillary astrocytes which have long processes rich in GFAP-positive filaments and are present in the white matter and, (2)
protoplasmic astrocytes with short processes and few GFAP-positive filaments and
mainly confined to the grey matter.

The cell processes of astrocytes form the background fibrillary meshwork called
'neuropil' (seen as pink background on the standard H&E stain).

Box 1.2 How to Identify an Astrocyte
Medium-size cell
Round or oval nucleus
Indistinct nucleolus
'Stellate' cell processes (seen with special stains such as PTAH; appear as
    pink background on H&E stain)

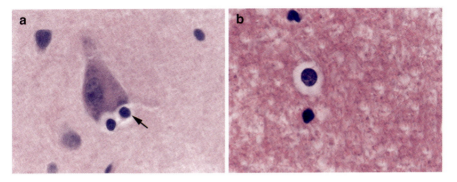

Fig. 1.4 (**a**) Oligodendrocytes (*arrow*) clustered around a neuron (satellite cells) and, (**b**) a typical oligodendrocyte with round nucleus and perinuclear halo in white matter. H&E stain

1.1.3   Oligodendrocytes

Oligodendrocytes are the myelin producing cells within the CNS. Oligodendrocytes are presumed to be derived from a common progenitor cell which also gives rise to neurons and depend on various regulatory factors for their differentiation and migration. The process of myelination is complex and relies on neuronal and axonal signals [2]. Each oligodendrocyte forms myelin segments on multiple axons. They are mainly present within the white matter along bundles of axons which they myelinate. Within the grey matter they are often seen around the cell body of neurons as 'satellite cells' (Fig. 1.4a). Oligodendrocyte, as the name implies, has fewer cytoplasmic processes compared to that of an astrocyte. These cell processes are not clearly visible on tissue sections. Therefore, these cells appear as naked dark round nuclei with 'perinuclear halo' or *'fried egg'* appearance (Fig. 1.4b, Box 1.3). This cytoplasmic clearing is not evident in intraoperative frozen sections or tissue which is rapidly fixed in formalin and is considered an artefact of delayed fixation. However, this is a very helpful feature in recognising a cell as being oligodendroglial in origin within a glial neoplasm.

> **Box 1.3 How to Identify an Oligodendrocyte**
> Small to medium-size cell
> Dark round nucleus
> Cytoplasmic clearing or 'perinuclear halo' or *'fried egg'* appearance

1.1.4   Schwann Cells

Schwann cells perform the function of electrically insulating axons of the peripheral nervous system. Unlike an oligodendrocyte, each Schwann cell myelinates only one axon. The cell processes of a Schwann cell wrap around an axon in

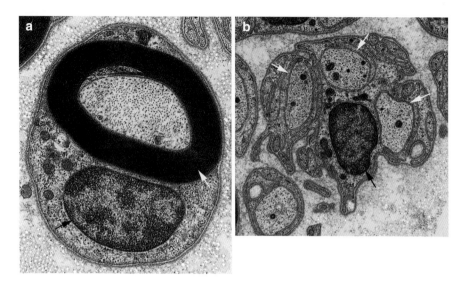

Fig. 1.5 (**a**) Ultrastructure of a peripheral nerve showing a large myelinated axon (*white arrow*) surrounded by a Schwann cell (*black arrow*) and, (**b**) Schwann cell (*black arrow*) wrapping three unmyelinated axons (*white arrows*) also referred to as a 'Remak cell'

multiple layers forming the myelin sheath (Fig. 1.5a). Large diameter axons are always myelinated whereas the small diameter axons can be myelinated or unmyelinated. Myelinated nerve fibers conduct electrical signals faster than unmyelinated fibers. Schwann cells also surround unmyelinated axons (Remak cell), with their cytoplasm wrapping around and isolating each axon from its neighbours (Fig. 1.5b). A Schwann cell also performs an important role in nerve regeneration after injury.

1.1.5 Ependyma

The ependymal cells form the lining of the ventricular system (in the brain) and central canal (in the spinal cord). They are believed to arise from ventricular (germinal) zone cells or radial glial cells. The ependyma plays an important role during early stages of brain development and in mature brain by supporting and protecting the subventricular (germinal) zone cells and also possibly in the circulation of cerebrospinal fluid within the ventricular system [3]. They are composed of a single layer of flattened or low cuboidal to columnar cells with apical cilia (Fig. 1.6). They have round to oval dark basal nucleus (Box 1.4).

Fig. 1.6 A layer of cuboidal ependymal cells with apical brush border/cilia (*arrow*). H&E stain

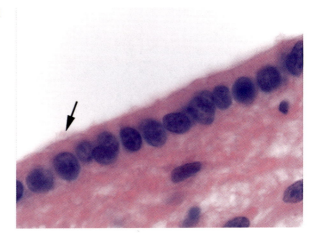

> **Box 1.4 How to Identify Ependyma**
> A single layer of flattened or low cuboidal or columnar epithelium
> Uniform round to oval dark basal nucleus
> Apical cilia

1.1.6   Microglia

Microglia are the resident cells of the immune system within the CNS. Therefore, in the strict sense they are not true glial cells but are derived from the bone marrow haematopoietic stem cells. They are now believed to have important role in synapse function and maintenance in a normal brain [4]. They are small cells (in comparison to macroglia- astrocytes, oligodendrocytes, and ependyma) with oval to elongated nuclei and contain numerous cytoplasmic processes. They are generally inconspicuous in normal healthy brains on H&E stain, but on close scrutiny can be seen as elongated/oval 'naked nuclei' and can be more clearly demonstrated by immunocytochemistry (Fig. 1.7; Box 1.5). They become more prominent in response to disease or injury. They can also transform into macrophages and help clean up the cellular debris and microorganisms.

> **Box 1.5 How to Identify Microglia**
> Small cell
> Elongated oval 'naked' nucleus
> Numerous cytoplasmic processes (not visible on H&E stain; can be seen with specific immunostains)

Fig. 1.7 Microglia or rod
cell with elongated
cytoplasmic processes
(*arrows*). HLA-DR
immunohistochemistry

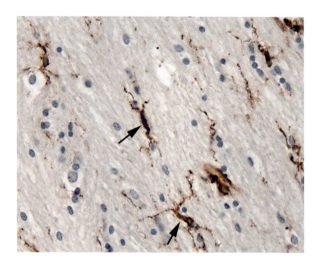

1.1.7 Supporting Tissues

The connective tissue which covers the brain and spinal cord is termed the 'meninges'. The dura mater (pachymeninges) forms the tough outermost layer, arachnoid mater the middle layer, and pia mater the innermost layer closely opposed to the brain and spinal cord surfaces. The arachnoid and pia mater are collectively termed leptomeninges. The tissues of the nervous system are richly supplied with blood vessels.

1.2 General Architecture of the Nervous System

1.2.1 Grey and White Matter

The grey matter is composed of cell bodies of neurons, dendrites and supporting glial cells. The microscopic structure of grey matter varies between different brain regions. The majority of cerebral cortex (also referred to as *'isocortex' or 'neocortex' or simply 'cortex'*) is made up of six distinct layers of neurons (Fig. 1.8a). The outer most layer is the paucicellular molecular layer without any neurons. Small granular neurons and large pyramidal neurons alternate in layers 2–6. The hippocampus shows three layer architecture (also termed *'archicortex'*). The cerebellar cortex also has only three layers which include the outer molecular layer, middle Purkinje cell layer and inner granular cell layer (Fig. 1.8b). In the brain, the grey matter is outside and the white matter is inside, whereas in the spinal cord the grey matter is deep inside and covered all around by white matter (Fig. 1.8c). Collections of neuronal cell bodies can also be found deep within the cerebrum and these form the deep grey nuclei (like basal

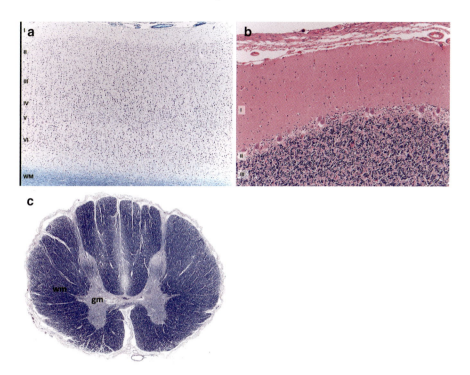

Fig. 1.8 (**a**) Six different layers of the cerebral cortex (LFB/CV stain), (**b**) three layers of the cerebellar cortex (H&E stain) and, (**c**) organisation of the spinal cord with grey matter on the inside and white matter on the outside (LFB/CV stain). *gm* grey matter, *wm* white matter

ganglia, thalamus, and dentate nucleus). The white matter is made up of bundles of myelinated axons. Bundles of myelinated axons which are responsible for similar function are termed as *'tracts'*. The midbrain, pons and medulla oblongata form the brainstem which contains the vital cardio-respiratory centres.

1.2.2 Peripheral Nerve

A nerve is a collection of axons (myelinated and unmyelinated) with other supporting cells including Schwann cells and fibroblasts. A peripheral nerve consists of three distinct compartments- the epineurium, perineurium and endoneurium. The epineurium is the outermost layer made up of fibroadipose connective tissue and also contains medium-sized blood vessels. The perineurium is the fibrous covering around a group of nerve fibers or axons and forms the nerve fascicle. The endoneurium is the innermost compartment containing individual myelinated (large or intermediate size) and unmyelinated (small) nerve fibers or axons along with Schwann cells and fibroblasts (Fig. 1.9a, b). (see Chap. 10 for more details).

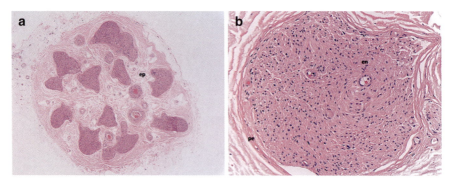

Fig. 1.9 Low (**a**) and high power (**b**) view of a normal peripheral nerve showing the three compartments- epineurium (*ep*), perineurium (*pe*) and the endoneurium (*en*). The endoneurium contains nerve fibers, Schwann cells, fibroblasts and blood vessels. H&E stain

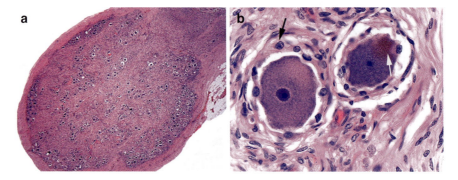

Fig. 1.10 Low (**a**) and high power (**b**) view of a dorsal root ganglion containing large neuronal cell bodies surrounded by satellite cells (*black arrow*). One of the neuron contains brown lipofuscin pigment in the cytoplasm (*white arrow*). H&E stain

1.2.3 Ganglia

A ganglion is a collection of neuronal cell bodies and their axons along with other supporting cells and lie outside the CNS (e.g. dorsal root ganglion of spinal nerves, ganglion of cranial nerves, sympathetic and parasympathetic ganglia). The dorsal root ganglia contain large pseudo unipolar neurons with their cell processes and surrounded by satellite cells (Fig. 1.10a, b). The autonomic ganglia contain smaller multipolar neurons.

1.2.4 Skeletal Muscle

Skeletal muscle is composed of compact fascicles of muscle fibres surrounded by the connective tissue, perimysium and epimysium. Each muscle fiber is polygonal or hexagonal in shape, has an outer cell membrane (sarcolemma) and inner cytoplasm (sarcoplasm). The nuclei are arranged at the periphery underneath the cell

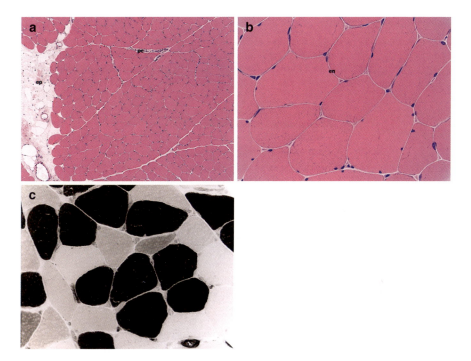

Fig. 1.11 (**a**, **b**) Low and high power microphotographs showing human skeletal muscle. The individual fibers are polygonal in shape with peripherally placed nuclei. H&E stain. (**c**) Shows two fiber types, the dark type 1 fibers and pale type 2 fibers. ATPase pH 4.4. *ep* epimysium, *pe* perimysium and, *en* endomysium

membrane (Fig. 1.11a, b). The sarcoplasm contains contractile proteins actin and myosin filaments. The connective tissue between each muscle fiber is scanty and is termed the endomysium. The perimysium is the connective tissue that surrounds groups of muscle fibers and forms a fascicle. Groups of fascicles are surrounded by epimysium. The muscle fibers are of two main types- type 1 (slow fibers) and type 2 (fast fibers) which can be recognised with histochemical stains (Fig. 1.11c). (see Chap. 9 for more details).

1.3 Commonly Used Stains in Neuropathology

1.3.1 Tinctorial Stains

A histopathologist or neuropathologist utilises several dyes to stain various tissue components thereby helping in the recognition and interpretation of abnormalities. The choice of stains used varies between different laboratories and also amongst pathologists. Table 1.1 lists some of the commonly used stains and their usefulness in diagnostic neuropathology.

Table 1.1 Tinctorial stains

Haematoxylin and Eosin (H&E)	Most commonly used stain in histopathology. Used for staining intra-operative smears, frozen sections, CSF cytospin preparations and formalin-fixed tissue. The haematoxylin stains nuclei blue and eosin stains the cytoplasm and cell processes pink. Most of the common pathologic features can be recognised using this stain
Toluidine blue	Rapid stain, used as an alternative to H&E stain, mainly for intraoperative smears. The nuclear details are better delineated with this stain. Also used to stain resin-embedded (semi-thin) sections of nerve and muscle
Cresyl violet or cresyl fast violet (CV/CFV)	Mainly used to study the morphology and distribution of neurons. Cresyl violet stains the Nissl substance dark purple or blue
Bielschowsky	This is a silver stain used to demonstrate axons. Axons are stained black. The stain can be performed on both frozen and paraffin sections. Can also be used to demonstrate senile plaques and neurofibrillary tangles in neurodegenerative diseases
Palmgren	Also a silver stain, which demonstrates axons as well as cell bodies of neurons. The axons and cell bodies of neurons are stained black
Luxol fast blue (LFB)	Stain used to demonstrate myelin within the CNS. Performed on formalin-fixed paraffin embedded tissue. Usually used in combination with Nissl stain (LFB/CV) or H&E (LFB/HE). Gives good contrast between grey and white matter and helps easy recognition of demyelinating lesions. Myelin is stained blue
Solochrome cyanin	Also a stain to demonstrate myelin, mainly used for peripheral nerves
Phosphotungstic acid haematoxylin (PTAH)	This demonstrates astrocytes and glial fibers. Before the advent of immunostains this stain was used as a glial lineage marker in brain tumours
Congo red	Stain used to demonstrate amyloid. Under polarised light, amyloid shows apple-green birefringence
Gram	Stain used to demonstrate bacteria. Gram positive bacteria appear blue/black
Periodic acid-Schiff (PAS)	This is used to demonstrate fungal organisms, glycogen in muscle, mucin in adenocarcinoma (in combination with Alcian blue) and basement membrane. PAS positive structures appear magenta coloured
Grocott	This is a silver stain used to identify fungal organisms which appear black
Ziehl-Neelsen (ZN)	This is a stain for *Mycobacterium tuberculosis,* an acid-fast bacillus. Positive organisms appear as slender red rods. A modification of this stain demonstrates *Mycobacterium leprae* (Wade-Fite stain)

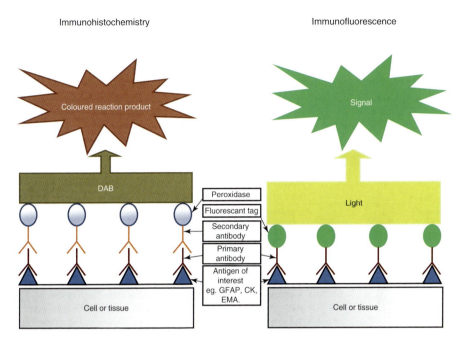

Fig. 1.12 Diagram showing the basic principles of immunohistochemistry (the peroxidise tagged to a secondary antibody binds to the antigen-antibody complex and converts DAB into a brown coloured reaction product) and immunofluorescence (a fluorophore tagged to a primary antibody binds to the antigen and emits fluorescent signal under UV light) techniques. *DAB* di-amino benzidine, *GFAP* glial fibrillary acidic protein, *CK* cytokeratin, *EMA* epithelial membrane antigen

1.3.2 Immunohistochemical Preparations

Immunohistochemistry is a technique of detecting tissue specific antigens by targeting them with specific antibodies. The resulting antigen-antibody interaction can be visualised in various ways. The commonly used detection method utilise antibody tagged with an enzyme called peroxidase (immunoperoxidase) which catalyses a colour producing reaction resulting in brown staining. Antibody tagged with a fluorophore (immunofluorescence) is also used widely in some laboratories (Fig. 1.12). Table 1.2 describes some of the most commonly used antibodies in diagnostic neuropathology.

Table 1.2 Antibodies used in diagnostic neuropathology

Glial fibrillary acidic protein (GFAP)	The intermediate filaments present in the cytoplasm of glial cells. This is widely used in identifying cells of glial lineage. It is strongly expressed in both reactive and neoplastic astrocytes and also variably in oligodendrocytes and ependyma
Synaptophysin	A major integral membrane protein of synaptic vesicles. This is a widely used marker of neuronal differentiation. The staining is localised to cell membrane and cytoplasm
Neu N	A neuronal marker and is localised to the nucleus
Neurofilament proteins (NFP)	A neuronal marker which is localised to cell bodies of neurons and their processes. It is particularly useful to detect native cell processes or axons within the tumours to distinguish infiltrative from non-infiltrative tumours
S-100	A protein expressed in cells derived from neural crest such as Schwann cells, glial cells and melanocytes. They are also expressed in chondrocytes, macrophages, adipocytes, myoepithelial cells, Langerhans cells, dendritic cells and keratinocytes
MIB-1 or Ki-67	Ki-67 is the antigen and MIB-1 is the antibody. This is the most commonly used marker for proliferating cells. High grade malignant tumours have a large proportion of proliferating cells and a high labelling index (expressed as %) compared to low grade or benign tumours
Epithelial membrane antigen (EMA)	The secretory product of MUC 1 gene and is expressed in a wide range of secretory epithelia and also the meninges
Cytokeratins (Cam5.2, MNF 116, AE1/AE3, CK7, CK20)	Intermediate cytoskeletal filaments present in the epithelial cells. They are useful in differentiating glial tumours from metastatic carcinomas
Thyroid transcription factor 1 (TTF-1)	Organ specific marker for tumours arising in the lung and thyroid gland
HMB-45, Melan-A	Markers of melanocytes and melanoma cells
Prostate specific antigen (PSA) and Prostate specific acid phosphatase (PSAP)	Organ specific markers used to detect carcinomas of prostate origin
Leucocyte Common Antigen (LCA/CD45)	Generic marker for all leucocytes
CD3	T-lymphocyte marker
CD20	B-lymphocyte marker
CD68	Monocyte/macrophage lineage marker
Beta-amyloid	This is the main component of most forms of CNS amyloid. It is widely used to detect amyloid in plaques and blood vessels in neurodegenerative diseases. Certain rare familial forms of amyloid disease can be negative with beta-amyloid
Beta-Amyloid Precursor Protein (Beta-APP)	Expressed in axonal injury due to various causes
Isocitrate dehydrogenase 1 (IDH-1)	Detects mutant IDH-1 in glial tumour cells. A significant proportion of diffuse gliomas are IDH-1 positive

References

1. Sofroniew MV, Vinters HV. Astrocytes: biology and pathology. Acta Neuropathol. 2010; 119(1):7–35.
2. Bradl M, Lassmann H. Oligodendrocytes: biology and pathology. Acta Neuropathol. 2010; 119(1):37–53.
3. Del Bigio MR. Ependymal cells: biology and pathology. Acta Neuropathol. 2010;119(1): 55–73.
4. Graeber MB, Streit WJ. Microglia: biology and pathology. Acta Neuropathol. 2010;119(1): 89–105.

Chapter 2
Basic Pathologic Reactions

Abstract This chapter deals with the ways in which the cellular constituents of the nervous system (neurons and glial cells) react to various insults. The severity and duration of the insult determine whether the final outcome is reversible or irreversible. Identification of these basic pathologic reactions helps the pathologist in making a diagnosis and also provides clues towards the aetiology of the pathological process.

Keywords Hypoxia • Ischaemia • Inclusions • Gliosis • Pathology

The cells which make up the nervous system and their supporting tissues can react to various insults in different ways. Many of these reactions are hard to recognise with naked eye examination and require microscopic analysis of the tissue. Sometimes, the morphology of these reactions provides clues about the aetiology of the pathological process.

2.1   Neurons

2.1.1   Neuronal Atrophy and Neuronal Loss

This is the end stage of irreversible neuronal injury. In atrophy, the cell body shrinks, cytoplasm shows diffuse basophilia and nucleus becomes dark or pyknotic. Neuronal loss is recognised by the accompanying increase in glial cells (gliosis), but sometimes may need detailed quantitative analysis. Atrophy and loss are commonly seen in aging and neurodegenerative diseases.

2.1.2   Hypoxic-Ischaemic Change

This is recognised by the presence of 'red neurons'- shrunken neurons with bright eosinophilic cytoplasm, dark, pyknotic nuclei and loss of nucleoli (Fig. 2.1). The red neurons are not specific to hypoxia/ischaemia, but can also be seen in

© Springer International Publishing Switzerland 2015
D.A. Hilton, A.G. Shivane, *Neuropathology Simplified: A Guide for Clinicians and Neuroscientists*, DOI 10.1007/978-3-319-14605-8_2

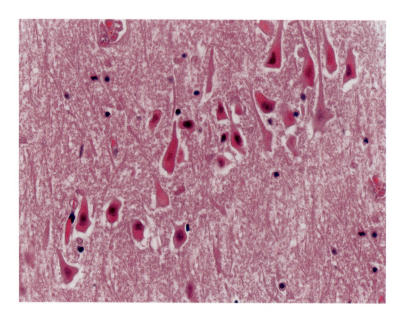

Fig. 2.1 The hippocampal pyramidal neurons showing hypoxic-ischaemic change (*red neurons*). H&E stain

hypoglycaemia and excitotoxic injury. Neurons in some locations are more vulnerable to hypoxic-ischaemic injury than others e.g. pyramidal neurons of hippocampus (Sommer sector or CA1), cortical neurons (layers 3 and 5) and cerebellar Purkinje neurons. The dead neurons may sometimes be encrusted with minerals such as calcium and iron (termed 'ferrugination'), commonly seen in infant brains with hypoxic-ischaemic injury.

2.1.3 Central Chromatolysis

This feature is recognised by the presence of a distended neuron with pale cytoplasm, loss of Nissl substance and eccentric location of the nucleus. This change is usually seen in lower motor neurons in the brainstem and spinal cord secondary to axonal damage. A similar change in neurons referred as 'ballooned or swollen neurons' can be seen in a wide variety of neurodegenerative, metabolic and developmental disorders.

2.1.4 Abnormal Inclusions

Accumulation of abnormal inclusions within a neuron (either in the cytoplasm or nucleus) (Fig. 2.2a–d) can be seen in various neurodegenerative diseases, metabolic diseases and viral infections (Table 2.1).

2.1.5 Axonal Alterations

Axonal swellings or spheroids are seen as a feature of axonal injury due to various insults, commonly trauma and ischaemia. The axonal swellings are best demonstrated in silver stains and by using immunohistochemistry for an antibody to beta-APP (Amyloid Precursor Protein) (Fig. 2.3). The axonal swellings have

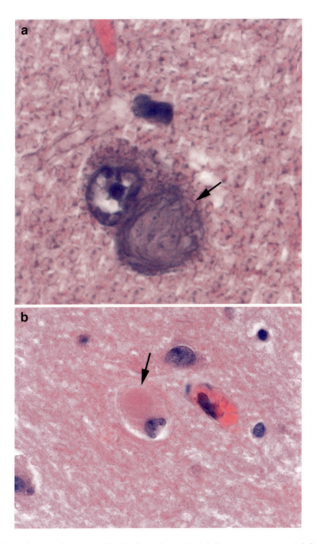

Fig. 2.2 Various abnormal neuronal inclusions (*arrow*). (**a**) Large neuron containing basophilic neurofibrillary (globose) tangle from a case of Alzheimer's disease, (**b**) cortical neuron showing eosinophilic Lewy body, (**c**) two Lewy bodies within a substantia nigra neuron from a case of Dementia with Lewy bodies, (**d**) anterior horn cell neuron containing eosinophilic beaded inclusion (Bunina body) from a case of motor neuron disease

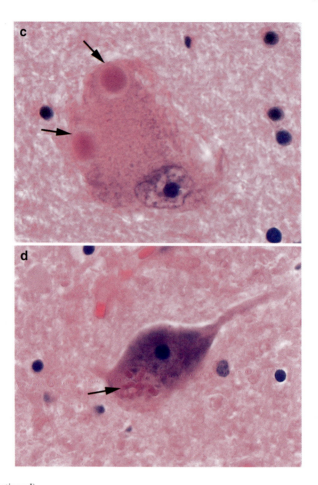

Fig. 2.2 (continued)

Table 2.1 Abnormal neuronal inclusions

Inclusion	Disease or association
Cowdry type A & B	Cytomegalovirus, Herpes, Measles, Poliomyelitis
Negri bodies	Rabies
Lewy bodies	Parkinson's disease, Dementia with Lewy bodies
Neurofibrillary tangles	Alzheimer's disease
Pick bodies	Pick's disease
Bunina bodies	Motor neuron disease
Lafora bodies	Myoclonic epilepsy
Polyglucosan bodies	Polyglucosan body disease

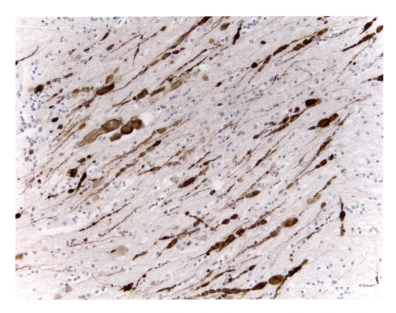

Fig. 2.3 A case of traumatic axonal injury showing numerous beta-APP positive axonal swellings

a characteristic distribution in cases of diffuse traumatic injury (see Chap. 13). A similar axonal swelling confined to the Purkinje neurons of cerebellum are termed 'axon torpedoes' and are seen in various cerebellar degenerations and also aging.

2.2 Astrocytes

2.2.1 Gliosis

Gliosis or astrogliosis refers to a process where astrocytes respond to injury by either increasing in size or number. In a normal brain tissue stained with routine H&E stain, astrocytes are visible as only naked nuclei. During the initial phase of injury, astrocytes increase in size and show prominent pink cytoplasm. These astrocytes are termed 'gemistocytic astrocytes' (means *'stuffed'* cells) (Fig. 2.4a). Gemistocytic astrocytes can also be a prominent feature in astrocytic tumours. In long standing or severe injury, the astrocytes proliferate and show prominent thin overlapping cytoplasmic processes rich in glial filaments. This is termed 'fibrillary

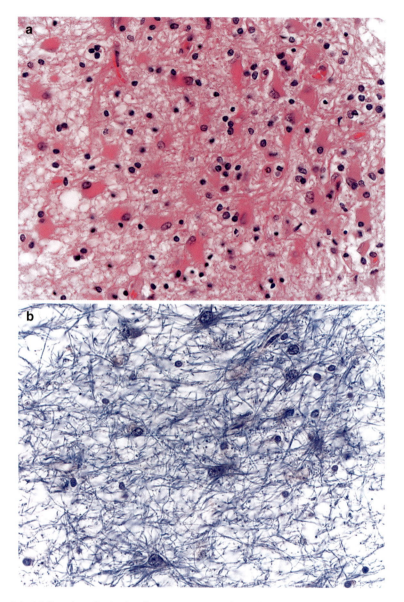

Fig. 2.4 (**a**) Reactive gliosis showing numerous gemistocytic astrocytes. H&E stain, (**b**) long-standing fibrillary gliosis. PTAH stain

gliosis' (Fig. 2.4b) which eventually leads to formation of a compact glial scar. This glial scar acts as a barrier and prevents entry of inflammatory cells and infectious agents [1]. 'Bergmann gliosis' refers to proliferation of Bergmann astrocytes whose cell bodies are located in the Purkinje cell layer of cerebellum and the cell processes extend into the molecular layer. 'Chaslin's gliosis' refers to gliosis in the subpial regions and is commonly seen in patients with long history of epilepsy. Gliosis can be identified using special stains such as PTAH or using immunohistochemistry for an antibody to GFAP. The impact of astrocytes on various CNS disorders is thought to be due to loss of its normal functions or gain of detrimental effects [1].

2.2.2 Alzheimer Type II Astrocyte

This is a special type of astrocyte seen mainly in metabolic conditions (such as Wilson disease and other forms of hepatic failure) where there is increase in blood ammonia levels. The astrocytes have clear or vesicular and irregular or multi-lobated nuclei and no visible cytoplasm. These cells are commonly seen within the deep grey nuclei, mainly in globus pallidus, and in brainstem.

2.2.3 Rosenthal Fibers

Rosenthal fibers are bright pink irregular, elongated or 'corkscrew' shaped structures within the cytoplasmic processes of astrocytes (Fig. 2.5a). They are seen in a wide variety of conditions including reactive gliosis, low-grade neoplasms (pilocytic astrocytoma, ganglion cell tumours, around long standing tumours such as craniopharyngioma or haemangioblastoma) and metabolic or genetic conditions such as Alexander's disease.

2.2.4 Eosinophilic Granular Bodies

Eosinophilic granular bodies or simply EGB's are rounded inclusions within the astrocyte cytoplasm containing granular pink material. They are mainly seen in low-grade tumours such as pilocytic astrocytoma or ganglion cell tumours.

2.2.5 Corpora Amylacea

These are rounded grey-blue cytoplasmic inclusions containing glucose polymers ('starch body'; intensely PAS-positive) mainly seen in the perivascular, subpial and subventricular regions (Fig. 2.5b). These inclusions accumulate in aging and also in a condition called 'Polyglucosan body disease'.

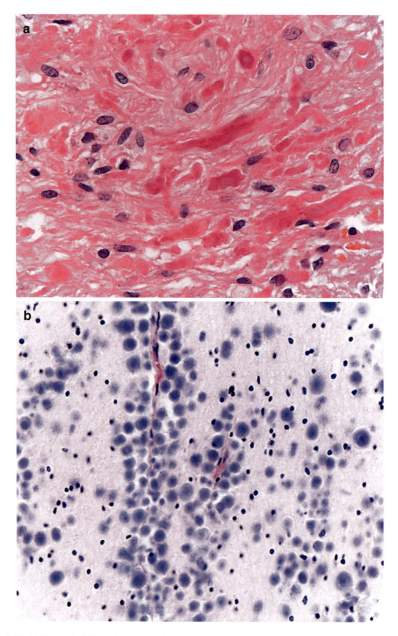

Fig. 2.5 (**a**) Rosenthal fibers in a case of pilocytic astrocytoma, (**b**) Corpora amylacea (*brain sand or starchy body*) within the neuropil. H&E stain

2.3 Oligodendrocytes

2.3.1 Demyelination

Oligodendrocytes are one of the most vulnerable cells of the CNS. Damage to oligodendrocytes results in demyelination i.e. loss of normal myelin with relative preservation of axons. The different patterns of white matter injury reflect different
mechanisms of oligodendrocyte damage such as primary oligodendrocyte damage,
damage to both oligodendrocyte and myelin or oligodendrocyte damage due to
energy deficiency [2]. Multiple sclerosis is the most common primary demyelinating
disorder where there is immunologically mediated myelin destruction. Demyelination
can also be caused by toxic and metabolic insults, viral infections and ischaemia.
Areas of demyelination can be identified as pale stained areas using special myelin
stains such as Luxol fast blue (Fig. 2.6). 'Dysmyelination' is the term used to describe
conditions where there is failure to form and maintain myelin (e.g. Leukodystrophies).

2.3.2 Inclusions

Oligodendrocytes can show typical ground glass nuclear inclusions when infected
with a *polyoma* virus called JC virus. This infection results in 'progressive multifocal
leukoencephalopathy or PML' and is common in immunosuppressed individuals.
Cytoplasmic oligodendroglial inclusions containing alpha-synuclein accumulate in
neurodegenerative conditions such as multiple system atrophy.

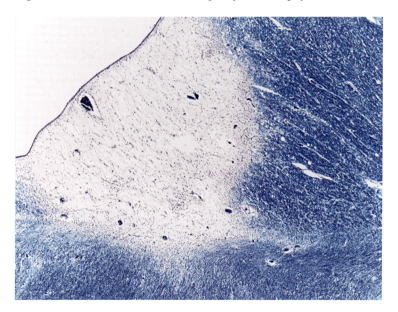

Fig. 2.6 A demyelinating plaque adjacent to the ventricle highlighted by a myelin stain. Luxol fast
blue stain

2.4   Ependyma

2.4.1   Atrophy

During ependymal atrophy, the cells lose their normal cuboidal or columnar profile and become flattened. This is seen in conditions such as hydrocephalus or cerebral atrophy.

2.4.2   Discontinuity

Discontinuity or breaks in ependymal lining is commonly seen in hydrocephalus, where the ventricle enlarges, and also in severe cerebral atrophy.

2.4.3   Granulations

When the ependymal lining is damaged, the astrocytes in the sub ependymal regions proliferate and form nodular protrusions into the ventricular cavity (Fig. 2.7). This is termed 'ependymal granulations' or 'granular ependymitis' (a misnomer as there is no inflammation associated with this lesion). This is a very non-specific marker of CNS injury and is observed in conditions such as hydrocephalus, viral infections and other non-infectious conditions.

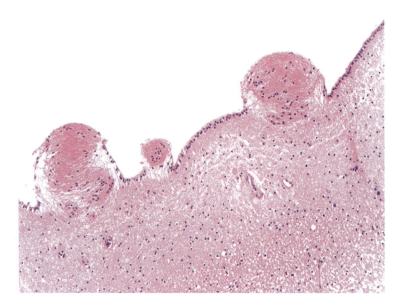

Fig. 2.7   Multiple ependymal granulations. H&E stain

2.5 Microglia

2.5.1 Diffuse Microglial Activation and Microglial Nodules

Diffuse microglial activation (Fig. 2.8a) is a very non-specific marker of CNS injury. Microglia can undergo either acute or chronic activation, both induced by signals from damaged neurons. In the acute phase, activated microglia provides support to

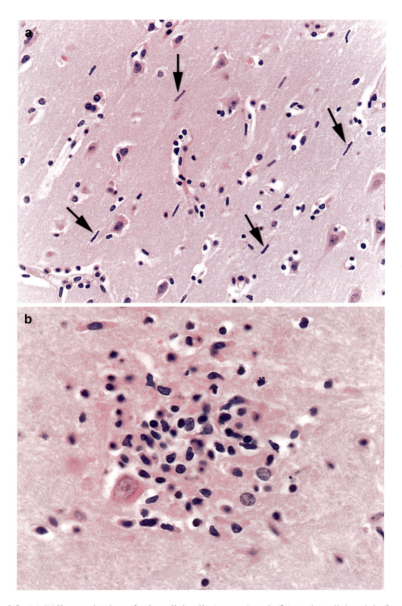

Fig. 2.8 (**a**) Diffuse activation of microglial cells (*arrows*) and, (**b**) a microglial nodule from a case of viral encephalitis. H&E stain

neurons and help in their recovery. Persistent or chronic activation results in degeneration of both microglia and neurons [3]. Microglial activation can be seen in a wide variety of conditions such as ischaemia, infections, inflammatory/immune-mediated diseases, neoplasms and neurodegeneration. Microglial nodules are considered hallmark of viral infections (Fig. 2.8b). Recent research focuses on the role of microglia in various neurodegenerative conditions [3].

References

1. Sofroniew MV, Vinters HV. Astrocytes: biology and pathology. Acta Neuropathol. 2010; 119(1):7–35.
2. Bradl M, Lassmann H. Oligodendrocytes: biology and pathology. Acta Neuropathol. 2010; 119(1):37–53.
3. Graeber MB, Streit WJ. Microglia: biology and pathology. Acta Neuropathol. 2010; 119(1):89–105.

Chapter 3
Requesting and Interpreting Pathological Tests

Abstract In order to maximise the chances of getting a diagnosis from a patient's specimen it is important that the correct tissue has been sampled, sent to the laboratory in the correct format and with the necessary clinical information. This chapter describes general and specific information about sending most specimen types to a laboratory to ensure that the pathologist has the best chance of providing a diagnosis. Particular care should be taken when undertaking muscle and nerve biopsies, which are very sensitive to artefactual damage which can limit their diagnostic value. In the investigation of a number of rare disorders specific samples and preservatives may be required, and in such cases prior liaison with the pathologist is advised. Interpretation of pathology reports should be undertaken with care, and in most cases this is best done in the context of a multidisciplinary team meeting.

Keywords Pathology test • Clinical information • Biopsy • CSF

In order to get the most out of any patient biopsy or fluid examination it is important that the correct sample is taken and sent to a laboratory with appropriate clinical information. If there is any doubt about what to sample, or how best to handle and send the specimen to the laboratory, always speak to the pathologist beforehand. It goes without saying that all specimens and specimen request forms should be clearly identified with patient details including name, date of birth, address and hospital reference number, to ensure that patient samples do not get mixed up (remember many laboratories receive thousands of samples each year and many of these will be from patients with similar names). The name and address of the doctor to whom the report is to be sent and the person taking the samples (if different), should also be included, along with relevant clinical information. For all specimens, if there is a likelihood of the patient harbouring a category 3 or 4 pathogen (e.g. HIV, hepatitis B or C, tuberculosis, CJD), then this should be clearly labelled on the form as 'high risk', so that the laboratory can take suitable precautions to minimise any danger to laboratory staff.

© Springer International Publishing Switzerland 2015   29
D.A. Hilton, A.G. Shivane, *Neuropathology Simplified: A Guide for Clinicians and Neuroscientists*, DOI 10.1007/978-3-319-14605-8_3

3.1 Neurosurgical Specimens

The majority of neurosurgical biopsies are taken from patients with tumours, and in order for the pathologist to correctly interpret the histology adequate clinical information should be provided (Box 3.1).

> **Box 3.1 Information to Include on Neurosurgical Request Forms**
> **Clinical history**, including neurological symptoms and signs, previous history of tumours.
> **Imaging findings**, including site, size and appearances of tumour, speed of growth, presence or absence of contrast enhancement.
> **Previous treatment,** including surgery, steroids, radiotherapy, preoperative embolisation and chemotherapy.
> **Family history** of tumours or other features to suggest a familial tumour syndrome.

Steroids may cause lymphomas to undergo marked reactive change, making diagnosis difficult and radiotherapy may result in secondary tumours (often many years later) and pathological changes such as radiation-induced necrosis. Preoperative embolization may cause changes that can be confused with malignancy such as mitoses and necrosis, particularly in meningiomas.

For large specimens (e.g. lobectomy) orientation may be important and in such cases identifying neurosurgical margins clearly with a suture, and adding this information to the request form, will aid in the pathologist being able to comment on involvement of various margins (almost always involved in diffuse gliomas). Most samples are placed in formalin before sending to the laboratory, however, with increasing frequency, genetic testing of tumour samples is important, and this is generally easier to undertake on fresh or frozen tissue. Depending on the type of genetic test undertaken, 'control' DNA from patient's peripheral blood lymphocytes may also be needed. Fresh tissue samples should be sent to the laboratory immediately to allow freezing before degradation occurs (unless rapid freezing facilities are available within operating theatre). It is important that the laboratory is informed in advance when sending fresh tissue, and depending on local staffing arrangements, these samples may need to be sent in normal working hours. In the case of brain biopsies taken from patients with rapidly progressive dementia where CJD is a possibility, fresh tissue is also required. In cases of rapidly progressive dementia the biopsy should include leptomeninges, and be taken from areas of contrast enhancement if possible, as this will increase the diagnostic yield of inflammatory disorders such as vasculitis. In the investigation of patients with suspected metabolic disorders, discussion with the laboratory is required beforehand. If an infective disorder is considered a possibility, separate specimens should be sent to the neuropathology and microbiology departments, latter generally requiring fresh tissue.

Intraoperative samples are often sent fresh to the laboratory where a rapid intraoperative diagnosis may affect surgical management (Box 3.2).

> **Box 3.2 Advantages of an Intraoperative Diagnosis**
> To provide a tumour diagnosis when this may affect the extent of surgical resection, or if the operative appearances do not match that expected from imaging.
> To confirm the presence of diagnostic material in stereotactic biopsies.
> To differentiate between tumour and infective/reactive conditions.
> To assess a surgical margin.
> To provide a diagnosis for the insertion of chemotherapeutic implants.
> To aid the immediate postoperative management.

In most cases this will involve sending a representative sample of tissue to the laboratory, although occasionally fluid may be useful e.g. for craniopharyngiomas. Generally intraoperative diagnoses take around 10–20 min to report and are very reliable (greater than 90 % accuracy), however, it is important that the laboratory is warned in advance of its arrival and that appropriate clinical information is provided as noted above.

Interpreting neurosurgical pathology reports for tumours is usually straightforward, as they are given a World Health Organisation (WHO) tumour classification and biological grade. It is important to note that the WHO tumour grade relates to the natural biological behaviour of the tumour without treatment, and not necessarily the prognosis with treatment. In addition, genetic subtyping of tumours has become important and can affect both prognosis and response to treatment, and this genetic information will become incorporated into future WHO tumour classification systems. There are a number of different methods for undertaking genetic analysis of tumour samples which may have differing advantages, and a particular difficulty with interpretation of brain tumour analysis is that the sample may not be 100 % tumour, e.g. diffuse gliomas, therefore interpretation should be done by, or in consultation with, the pathologist.

Pathology reports may not be conclusive: the biopsy may show reactive changes which could imply reactive change within a tumour (e.g. lymphoma treated with steroids) or a non-neoplastic condition; it may show necrotic tissue which is non-diagnostic and should not necessarily be interpreted as a malignant tumour as other conditions may also cause necrosis (e.g. infarcts and abscesses); or it may show hypercellular tissue, and it is not always possible to determine whether the cells are infiltrating tumour cells or reactive cells. If the report concludes infiltrating glial tumour, then the tumour grading and subtyping may not be reliable, particularly as there may be areas of higher grade tumour which were not included in the biopsy. Proper interpretation of the pathology is always best undertaken as part of a multidisciplinary team meeting where the clinical findings, intraoperative findings and imaging can be discussed alongside the pathology and genetic findings.

3.2 Muscle and Nerve Biopsies

In addition to the clinical history and neurological findings, it is important that the biopsy is taken from a clinically affected area. In the case of muscle biopsies the pattern of weakness (e.g. proximal and/or distal) should be noted on the request form and the sample should be taken from a muscle that is clinically involved, but not so severely that it will result in end stage disease pathology. Sometimes MRI imaging of muscle may help in identifying a clinically affected muscle group for sampling. The clinical information should include results of electromyography, serum creatinine kinase levels, recent immunosuppressive treatment, and any additional relevant clinical findings such as skin rashes, involvement of the central nervous system, heart or respiratory system. It is also useful to include a detailed family history and the results of any genetic testing undertaken. Similarly with nerve biopsies it is important that the results of nerve conduction studies are included along with a detailed family history and the results of any genetic investigations. Most nerve biopsies are undertaken from sensory nerves (e.g. sural nerve, superficial peroneal nerve or superficial radial nerve), and there should be either clinical or electrical evidence of involvement of the relevant nerve that is sampled.

Muscle and nerve biopsies are generally sent to the laboratory fresh (unless by prior agreement with the laboratory). They should arrive in the laboratory as soon as possible after removal (within 20 min), and the laboratory should be informed in advance so that they can prepare the relevant reagents required for freezing and fixing the samples. Normally a small part of the muscle or nerve biopsy is fixed in glutaraldehyde for more detailed examination, including electron microscopy. Nerve biopsies should be removed with extreme care by the surgeon undertaking the procedure, as artefacts are very common if the sample is cauterised, stretched or kinked. Local anaesthetic should not be injected directly into the muscle group being sampled, but only as deep as the fascia. Interpretation of the findings of muscle and nerve biopsies is best undertaken at a multidisciplinary team meeting where the clinical information can be presented along with neurophysiological findings.

3.3 Cerebrospinal Fluid

It is important that where different laboratory analyses are required the sample is divided into separate specimen pots and sent to the relevant sections of the pathology laboratory. Usually different areas of the laboratory will be responsible for protein analysis, microbiological assessment or assessment of the presence of cells and their nature. When taking CSF samples to look for malignant cells, an adequate volume should be sent (usually at least 5 ml), and it should arrive in the laboratory promptly during normal working hours, so that it can be prepared immediately to optimise cellular preservation. Sending a larger volume will allow more fluid to be examined for cells, and also additional tests such as immunohistochemistry, to allow reliable subtyping of any cells present.

3.4   Skin Biopsies

These may be taken for a number of different reasons including looking for a small fibre neuropathy, Parkinson's disease, hereditary disorders such as CADASIL, Lafora body disease, Kuf's disease, Niemann-Pick disease type C and Batten's disease. For each of these different investigations particular areas of skin may need to be sampled, and different preservatives are required including formalin, glutaraldehye and Zamboni's fixative. In some cases fresh tissue is required and it is therefore important to discuss these biopsies in advance with the pathologist.

3.5   Other Samples

Temporal artery biopsies for giant cell arteritis should be placed in formalin intact, and the diagnostic sensitivity is greater if a longer sample is removed (>1 cm), and if bilateral sampling is undertaken. In certain rare paediatric disorders samples of blood, hair or urine may be required. Please consult with the laboratory in such cases.

Chapter 4
Vascular Diseases

Abstract Diseases affecting the blood vessels of the CNS constitute an important group and are associated with significant morbidity and mortality. This chapter starts with a basic discussion of CNS vascular anatomy before going into specific diseases. Atherosclerosis is the most common vascular disease and is a major cause for stroke and vascular dementia. The majority of vascular diseases are sporadic and multifactorial, but a few rare hereditary forms also occur such as CADASIL and familial amyloid angiopathies. Vasculitides form an important group of treatable conditions which also pose considerable diagnostic challenge for both clinician and pathologist. The end result of most vascular disease is ischaemia, infarction or haemorrhage.

Keywords Blood vessel • Malformation • Inflammation • Infarction • Haemorrhage

The brain is a highly metabolically active organ and depends largely on aerobic metabolism for its survival with very little capacity for anaerobic metabolism. This high demand is reflected in the cerebral blood flow which is 20 % of the cardiac output, even though the brain makes up only 2 % of the body weight. The blood vessels ensure delivery of a continuous supply of important nutrients like oxygen and glucose to tissues of the nervous system. Even a short interruption of blood flow to the brain results in disastrous consequences. The diseases which affect the nervous system vasculature can cause either (1) global or focal interruption to blood flow leading to ischaemia and infarction, or (2) leakage or rupture of blood vessels leading to haemorrhage.

4.1 Vascular Anatomy

4.1.1 Arterial Supply

Two major pairs of arteries supply blood to the brain, the internal carotid arteries (anterior circulation) and vertebral arteries (posterior circulation). The anterior circulation carries roughly 70–80 % of blood supply and the posterior circulation the remaining 20–30 %. The internal carotid arteries (ICA) branch off from the common carotid arteries in the neck and enter the cranial cavity. They pass through

© Springer International Publishing Switzerland 2015   35
D.A. Hilton, A.G. Shivane, *Neuropathology Simplified: A Guide for Clinicians and Neuroscientists*, DOI 10.1007/978-3-319-14605-8_4

the cavernous sinus and then divide into two branches, the middle cerebral arteries (MCA) and anterior cerebral arteries (ACA). The vertebral arteries (VA) arise from the subclavian and brachiocephalic arteries and pass through the transverse foramina of C1-C6 vertebrae and enter the cranial cavity via the foramen magnum. The largest branch of VA is posterior inferior cerebellar artery (PicA). Along the ventral surface of the brainstem the two VA join to form the basilar artery which then divides into two posterior cerebral arteries (PCA). The two ACA are joined by anterior communicating artery (AComA). The PCA join with the ICA via posterior communicating arteries (PComA) to complete the circle of Willis (Fig. 4.1). There is considerable anatomical variation in the arteries forming the circle of Willis. Anastomoses within the circle of Willis allow collateral supply of blood in the event of arterial blockage.

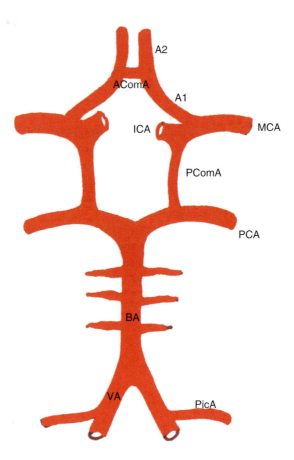

Fig. 4.1 Diagram of Circle of Willis showing all the major branches. *A1, A2* segments of anterior cerebral artery, *AComA* anterior communicating artery, *MCA* middle cerebral artery, *ICA* internal carotid artery, *PCA* posterior cerebral artery, *PComA* posterior communicating artery, *BA* basilar artery, *VA* vertebral artery, and *PicA* posterior inferior cerebellar artery

The branches of the MCA supplies most of the lateral aspect of the brain and deeper structures like striatum, internal capsule, hippocampus, amygdala, optic radiation and choroid plexus. Occlusion of MCA or one of its key perforating branches produces the 'classic hemiplegic stroke' affecting the putamen and internal capsule. The ACA supplies the medial aspect of frontal and parietal lobes, anterior limb of internal capsule and corpus callosum. The branches of PCA supply the inferior and medial aspects of temporal and occipital lobes, thalamus and posterior limb of internal capsule. Branches from the VA, basilar artery and PCA supply the entire brainstem and cerebellum.

The blood supply to the spinal cord is by the branches of VA- the two posterior spinal arteries (PSA) (posterior third of the cord) and a single anterior spinal artery (ASA) (anterior two-thirds of the cord) (Fig. 4.2a, b). The cord is also reinforced by radicular arteries arising from segmental vessels including the ascending cervical, intercostal and lumbar arteries.

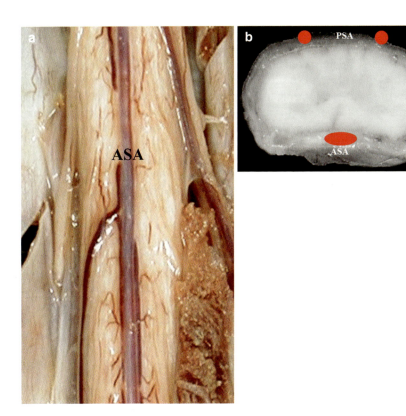

Fig. 4.2 (**a, b**) Vascular supply of spinal cord. *ASA* anterior spinal artery, *PSA* posterior spinal artery

4.1.2 Venous Drainage

The venous drainage is through superficial and deep veins. The superficial veins in the subarachnoid space empty into the venous sinuses. The upper part of the brain drains into superior sagittal sinus, the middle part into the cavernous sinus and the lower part into the transverse sinus. The deep veins drain into the great cerebral vein of Galen and through straight sinus empties into the transverse sinus. The blood from transverse sinuses drains to sigmoid sinus, internal jugular vein and then to the heart through brachiocephalic vein and superior vena cava.

The anterior and posterior spinal veins drain blood from the cord into the vertebral venous plexus. The blood from plexus drains into lumbar veins, azygos and hemiazygos veins.

4.2 Diseases Affecting the Blood Vessels

4.2.1 Atherosclerosis

Atherosclerosis is the most common vascular disease and mainly affects large and medium-sized muscular and elastic arteries. It is also the most important cause for ischaemic stroke. In the intracranial compartment, the internal carotid and basilar arteries are the most severely affected. The risk factors for atherosclerosis include-increasing age, male gender, hyperlipidaemia, gene polymorphisms (*ABCA1*, *MMP-3, IL-6 genes*) [1–3], hypertension, cigarette smoking and diabetes.

Over the years several theories have been postulated for the formation of the atherosclerotic plaque or atheroma ('*Atheroma*' = Greek word for '*Gruel*'). These include-(1) cellular proliferation within the intima, (2) organisation and growth of thrombi, and (3) vascular injury or response to injury theory. The latter is currently the favoured hypothesis. The endothelium can become dysfunctional or injured by various factors such as mechanical, excess lipid, toxins, bacterial and viral infections, haemodynamic stress and immune reactions. The injured endothelium attracts monocytes circulating in the blood and also the smooth muscle cells from the media into the intima. Lipids also accumulate within the vessel wall during this process. The damaged endothelium release growth factors which help in the proliferation of smooth muscle cells eventually culminating in plaque formation (Table 4.1). The plaque can undergo disruption and precipitate thrombus formation that can further obstruct blood flow.

4.2.2 Small Vessel Disease

As the name implies, small vessel disease (SVD) affects mainly the small perforating arteries or arterioles, venules and capillaries. The compromise of blood supply due to SVD can result in distinct disorders which include- lacunar infarcts (small

Table 4.1 Morphology of plaques

Lesion	Description
Fatty streak	Earliest lesion (even seen in children as young as 10 years). Appear as yellow flat lesions. Contain lipid-filled foam cells. Do not cause any disturbance to blood flow.
Fibrofatty plaque (Fig. 4.3)	Appear as white to pale yellow raised lesion containing lipid in the core and covered by firm white fibrous cap. These lesions impinge on the vascular lumen, are usually eccentric and patchy along the length of the vessel.
Complicated plaque	A fibrofatty plaque which shows evidence of rupture, ulceration or erosion, haemorrhage, thrombus formation or aneurysmal dilatation.

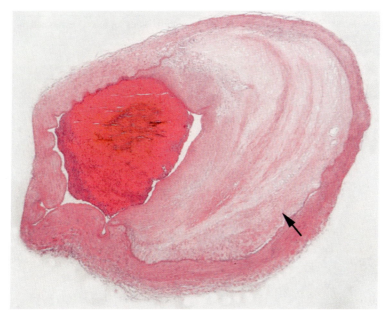

Fig. 4.3 A large artery showing intimal fibro-fatty atheromatous plaque (*arrow*) and luminal narrowing. H&E stain

infarcts ≤1.0 cm), vascular dementia and primary non-traumatic parenchymal brain haemorrhage. The risk factors associated with SVD include age, diabetes and hypertension. The MRI scan of brain typically shows symmetric, multifocal abnormality within the white matter and basal ganglia. Small blood vessels in the brain can be affected in vast number of diseases such as inflammatory, infective, toxic and hereditary disorders, but the three common conditions include arteriolosclerosis (including Binswanger's disease), cerebral amyloid angiopathy (CAA) and cerebral autosomal dominant arteriopathy with sub-cortical infarcts and leukoencephalopathy (CADASIL). Binswanger's disease is a sporadic condition affecting elderly hypertensive patients. The pathology is characterised by arteriolosclerosis and multiple white matter infarcts. Table 4.2 describes the pathological features of SVD.

Table 4.2 Pathological features of small vessel disease

Lesion	Description
Atherosclerosis	Atheromas similar to those seen in the larger blood vessels. Because of the small size of the vessels affected, even a small atheroma can compromise the lumen considerably.
Fibrinoid necrosis and Lipohyalinosis	Fibrinoid necrosis refers to the early stage where the leakage of blood–brain barrier results in deposits of plasma proteins including fibrin in the vessel wall. The vessels at this stage are vulnerable to rupture. At a later stage, the wall will be replaced by acellular fibrosis with little or no lipid termed '*lipohyalinosis*'.
Arteriolosclerosis (Fig. 4.4)	Hyaline thickening of the arterioles. Commonly associated with clinical vascular dementia.
Micro-aneurysms	Now believed to be 'complex tortuosities' of blood vessels and the causation is unclear [4].

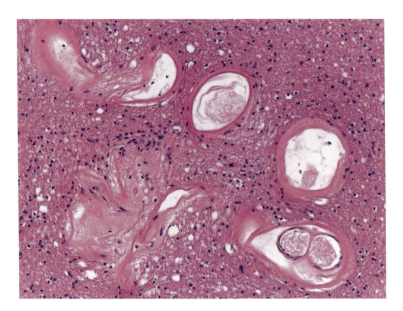

Fig. 4.4 Small blood vessels within the white matter showing prominent thickening and hyalinisation suggestive of small vessel disease. H&E stain

4.2.3   Amyloid Angiopathy

The cerebral amyloid angiopathy (CAA) is characterised by the deposition of fibrillar amyloid protein (Box 4.1) in the walls of blood vessels of the brain and meninges. There are several different amyloidogenic proteins (Table 4.3).

The sporadic form of CAA is more common than hereditary CAA subtypes, and is composed of Aβ amyloid. Sporadic Aβ-CAA is the most common cause of lobar haemorrhage in the elderly. The prevalence of CAA is high in patients with Alzheimer's disease (>90 %) and they also share some of the risk factors (genetic polymorphisms in ApoE, PS1, α-1 anti-chymotrypsin, neprilysin) [5]. Some of the other conditions associated with Aβ deposition include Downs syndrome, Dementia pugilistica and vascular malformations.

Table 4.3 The amyloid angiopathies

Disease	Gene involved/precursor protein	Type of amyloid
Sporadic Aβ-CAA (commonly associated with sporadic Alzheimer's disease)	APP/Amyloid precursor protein	Aβ
Hereditary Aβ CAA (Dutch and Flemish types, Familial Alzheimer's disease)	APP/Amyloid precursor protein	Aβ
Hereditary cerebral haemorrhage with amyloid angiopathy- Icelandic type	CYST C/Cystatin C	ACys
Familial amyloidosis- Finnish type	GEL/Gelsolin	AGel
Familial British Dementia	BRI2/ABri	ABri
Familial Danish Dementia	BRI2/ADan	ADan
Familial Amyloidotic Polyneuropathy/ Meningovascular amyloidosis	TTR/Transthyretin	ATTR
Prion protein CAA	PRNP	APrP

Box 4.1 Characteristics of Amyloid
Misfolded protein which acquires β-pleated secondary structure
Highly insoluble
Binds stains such as Congo red (apple-green birefringence under polarised light) and Thioflavin-S or T (fluorescence)
Can be demonstrated by immunohistochemistry using an antibody to β-amyloid or other amyloidogenic proteins

The macroscopic examination of brain with sporadic Aβ-CAA may show lobar haemorrhages mainly in the frontal or fronto-parietal lobes. Cerebellar haemorrhages are infrequent. There may be changes of associated Alzheimer's disease, petechial haemorrhages and small infarcts in the grey or white matter. The small to medium-sized arteries/arterioles in the leptomeninges and cortex are preferentially affected. The amyloid deposition is more severe in the posterior cerebrum (parietal and occipital lobes). The affected blood vessels appear rounded and thickened, show deposition of amyloid within the tunica media and adventitia (Fig. 4.5a). The amyloid can be confirmed to be Aβ using immunohistochemistry (Fig. 4.5b). In some cases, the Aβ-laden blood vessel can show giant cell/granulomatous reaction which is termed 'Aβ-related angiitis'.

4.2.4   Hereditary Vascular Diseases

CADASIL is the acronym for Cerebral Autosomal Dominant Arteriopathy with Subcortical Infarcts and Leukoencephalopathy, which was first described by van Bogaert in 1955. The defective gene was identified in 1996 to be Notch3 located on chromosome 19. This is a slowly progressive vascular disease equally affecting males and females with onset of stroke before the age of 30 years; the clinical presentation peaks around 40–50 years of age. The classic symptoms include- migraine with

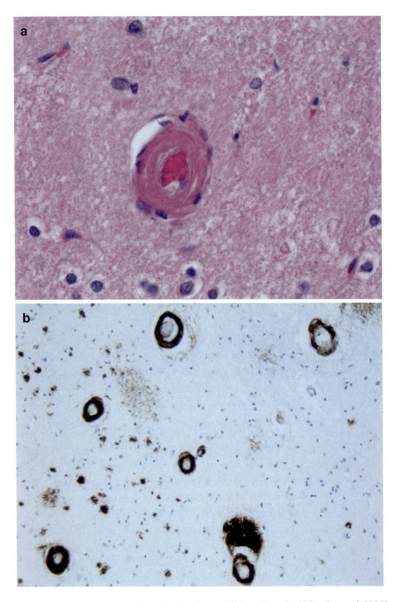

Fig. 4.5 (**a**) Cerebral amyloid angiopathy showing a thickened cortical blood vessel, H&E stain, (**b**) cortical blood vessels showing beta-amyloid deposition within their walls, Beta-amyloid immunohistochemistry

aura, ischaemic attacks, psychiatric symptoms, cognitive decline and dementia and rarely seizures. Hyperintensities on T2 weighted and flair MRI within the tempo-ral poles is diagnostic of CADASIL. This disease affects small and medium-sized arteries, and rarely veins, of almost all organs. Therefore, skin biopsy is very useful for the diagnosis of CADASIL. The blood vessels become markedly thickened and fibrotic with accumulation of basophilic, PAS-positive granular material within the tunica media. There is accompanying degeneration of vascular smooth muscle cells. In the brain, the vessels in the leptomeninges and white matter are preferentially affected. The narrowing of vascular lumina results in ischaemic lesions mainly in the white matter, deep grey structures, brainstem and rarely in the spinal cord, but spares the cortical grey matter. The ultrastructural examination of the arteries reveals destruction of smooth muscle cells and accumulation of granular osmiophilic material (GOM), pathognomonic of this disease. An antibody against the extracellular domain of Notch3 is available and may be useful in making a diagnosis [6]. Majority of CADASIL cases demonstrate missense point mutations in the Notch3 gene with more than 130 different mutations identified so far. The pathogenesis of this disease is still unclear, but it is thought that the mutated Notch3 protein accumulation is likely to exert a toxic effect.

CARASIL (Cerebral Autosomal Recessive Arteriopathy with Subcortical Infarcts and Leukoencephalopathy) is another small vessel arteriopathy with recessive inheritance, orthopaedic problems (such as herniation of intervertebral disc, kyphosis, and ossification of spinal ligaments) and similar MRI features and infarcts as in CADASIL. This disease is also termed 'Maeda syndrome' [7]. This disease is extremely rare and has been reported mainly from Japan. The onset is between 20 and 45 years and more common in males. Multiple small foci of softening are noted within the cerebral white matter, basal ganglia and brainstem along with small vessel changes such as intimal thickening, destruction of elastic lamina and smooth muscle and thinning of adventitia. There is not much information about the gene defect in this disease and a reliable diagnosis using skin biopsy is not available yet.

4.2.5   Vasculitides

The term 'vasculitis' refers to inflammation of the blood vessel wall with associated necrosis or destruction of the vessel wall (Fig. 4.6). Vasculitis affecting CNS blood vessels can have several different aetiologies (Table 4.4). Both clinically and pathologically they can be quite challenging to diagnose. Various classifications have been proposed based on pathology, the type of blood vessel (calibre) or presumed aetiology.

Giant cell or temporal arteritis (GCA) is the commoner of the four primary CNS vasculitides and mainly affects the extracranial arteries of the head and neck. The involvement of superficial temporal and ophthalmic arteries is well recognised but in a small proportion of cases the carotid and vertebral arteries may also be involved. Clinically, affected patients are usually females over the age of 50 years and present with headache, temporal swelling and tenderness, transient or permanent blindness or stroke. The disease is commonly associated with polymyalgia rheumatica. The cause of GCA is not known but is presumed to be a cell mediated immune injury to an unknown antigen. The histology of the temporal artery shows

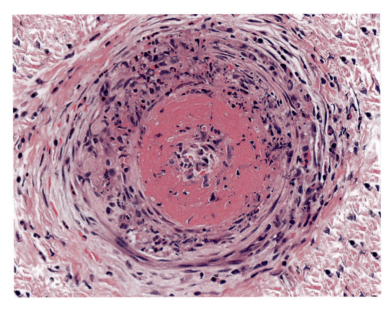

Fig. 4.6 Vasculitis in a patient with Sjogren's syndrome. There is intimal thickening, fibrinoid necrosis and transmural inflammation consisting of lymphocytes and a few eosinophils. H&E stain

Table 4.4 The different types of CNS vasculitides

Non-infectious	Infectious
Primary vasculitis involving the CNS	*Bacterial vasculitis*
Giant cell or temporal arteritis (GCA)	Streptococcus, Mycobacteria, Spirochaetes (Treponema, Borrelia)
Primary angiitis of CNS (PACNS)	*Viral vasculitis*
Takayasu's arteritis	Herpes zoster, HIV, Hepatitis B & C, EBV
Kawasaki's disease	*Fungal vasculitis*
Aβ-related angiitis	Aspergillus, Candida, Coccidioides, Mucor sp.
Vasculitis due to systemic disease	*Other microbes*
Systemic lupus erythematosus (SLE), polyarteritis nodosa (PAN), Wegener's granulomatosis, Churg-Strauss syndrome, Sjogren's syndrome, Behcet's syndrome, Rheumatoid arthritis.	Protozoa, Mycoplasma, Rickettsia sp.
Vasculitis associated with malignancy	
Hodgkin and non-Hodgkin lymphoma	
Drug-induced vasculitis	
Cocaine, Amphetamines, Phenylpropanolamine	

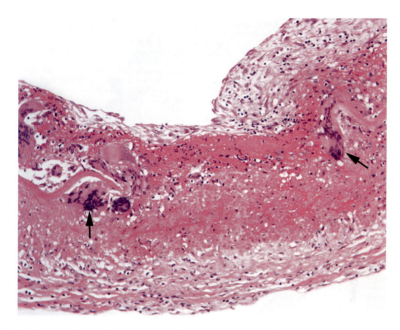

Fig. 4.7 Giant cell arteritis showing multinucleated giant cells (*arrows*) and sparse chronic inflammation within the blood vessel wall. H&E stain

a granulomatous inflammation with T-lymphocytes, epithelioid macrophages, occasional eosinophils and multinucleated giant cells of foreign body or Langhans' type (Fig. 4.7). The inflammation spreads from the outer adventitia into the inner layers. The lack of giant cells or complete absence of inflammation does not exclude GCA as the disease can be very focal and patchy. Therefore, a decent length of temporal artery (>1 cm) biopsy is recommended and the tissue is examined for inflammation by sectioning at multiple levels. In later stages, there is marked intimal thickening, destruction of elastic lamina, calcification, thickened or fibrotic media and adventitia, compromising the vascular lumen and resulting in thrombosis or infarction. The disease responds favourably to corticosteroid therapy.

Primary angiitis of CNS (PACNS) previously termed 'Granulomatous angiitis of CNS' or 'Isolated angiitis of CNS' is a rare entity and is a diagnosis of exclusion. Patients with PACNS do not have any systemic inflammatory disease, infections, neoplasm or drug exposure. Patients present with non-specific symptoms which include headache, focal or non-focal neurological deficits and encephalopathy. There are no diagnostic blood tests for PACNS. CSF analysis may show moderate pleocytosis and elevated protein levels. Brain imaging findings include multiple infarcts, meningeal enhancement or diffuse white matter changes. Angiography may show alternate areas of stenosis and ectasia in multiple vascular distributions. Brain biopsy remains the gold standard for the diagnosis of PACNS. The temporal pole from non-dominant hemisphere (approximately 1 cm^3 in size and should include the leptomeninges) is the preferred site in the absence of focal lesions. The

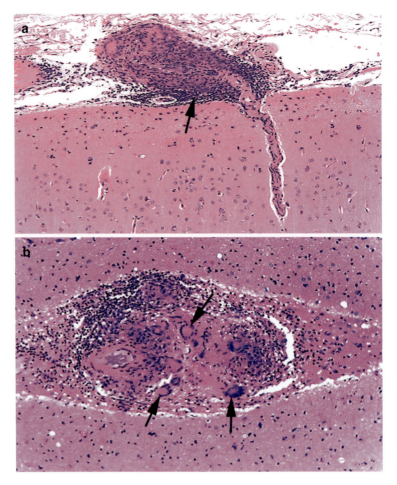

Fig. 4.8 (**a**) Brain biopsy from a patient with primary angiitis of CNS (PACNS) showing lympho-cytes around a leptomeningeal artery (*arrow*), and (**b**) granuloma with multinucleated giant cells (*arrows*). H&E stain

pathology shows granulomatous, necrotising or lymphocytic inflammation in and around the walls of small leptomeningeal and intracerebral vessels (Fig. 4.8a, b). The vasculitis can be focal and segmental and therefore, a negative biopsy does not necessarily exclude PACNS. The disease once considered fatal can now be treated with a favourable outcome using aggressive immunosuppression.

4.2.6 Vascular Malformations

Vascular malformations arise as a result of disordered mesodermal differentia-tion during embryonic life. They carry a significant risk of intracranial bleeding. McCormick in 1966 [8] proposed a simple classification which included five

Table 4.5 Classification of CNS vascular malformations (simplified)

Cerebral and spinal cord parenchyma
Arteriovenous malformation (AVM)
Venous angioma and varix (varicose vein)
Capillary telangiectasia
Cavernous angioma
Combined: capillary + cavernous; cavernous + venous
Leptomeninges
Arteriovenous malformation
Venous angioma and varix
Dura
Arteriovenous malformation
Cavernous angioma
Vein of Galen malformations

types- (1) telangiectasia, (2) varix, (3) cavernous angioma, (4) venous angioma and, (5) arterio-venous malformation (AVM). This classification has now been updated to include not only developmental lesions but also a few acquired vascular lesions; location, morphology and aetiology (Table 4.5) [9].

Majority of vascular malformations are sporadic, however, familial cavernous angiomas linked to genes *CCM 1–3* (*cerebral cavernous malformation 1–3*) have been described.

AVM (Figs. 4.9a and 4.10a), the most dangerous of all the vascular malformations show abnormal arteries and veins communicating directly without any intervening capillary network. They are typically wedge-shaped lesions with base near the leptomeninges and apex within the parenchyma. The intervening and surrounding parenchyma may show chronic gliosis, old or fresh haemorrhage. An elastic van Gieson (EVG) stain is useful to delineate arteries and veins. *Venous angiomas* (Fig. 4.9b) are composed of one or more dilated venous channels, but no arteries. A *varix* is a single dilated and tortuous vein. Venous angiomas are the commonest malformation seen at autopsy. Typical sites include brain parenchyma and the subarachnoid space of lower thoracic spinal cord. *Cavernous angiomas* (Figs. 4.9c and 4.10b) are well defined lesions containing closely-packed, thin-walled blood vessels with minimal or no intervening brain or spinal cord parenchyma. They are common in the subcortical white matter, pons and external capsule region. Temporal lobe lesions can cause intractable epilepsy. *Capillary telangiectases* (Fig. 4.9d) is a collection of dilated capillaries with intervening brain parenchyma. They are usually small and incidental lesions commonly found in the pons, but can also occur in other regions of brain and spinal cord.

4.2.7 Aneurysms

Aneurysm is defined as 'a localised and persistent dilatation of an artery'. Within the CNS they can be of various types and include- saccular (berry) aneurysm, mycotic/infectious, fusiform, atherosclerotic and dissecting aneurysms. *Saccular or*

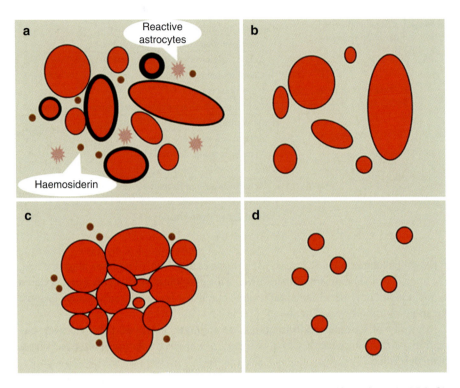

Fig. 4.9 Schematic diagram showing the common types of vascular malformation. (**a**) AVM, (**b**) venous angioma, (**c**) cavernous angioma, (**d**) capillary telangiectases

berry aneurysms (BA) (Fig. 4.11a, b) are the commonest, usually presents with rupture and represent the most important cause of spontaneous (non-traumatic) subarachnoid haemorrhage. BA can be multiple and familial in a small proportion of patients. BA arise at or close to the bifurcation of the arteries where the haemodynamic stress is more. Almost 90 % of BA occur in the anterior circulation and only in 10 % of cases involve the posterior circulation. However, in children, the posterior circulation is involved in 40–45 % of cases. BA should be suspected in patients who die from spontaneous subarachnoid haemorrhage. The distribution of haemorrhage can sometimes predict the site of BA. The EVG stain may demonstrate focal disruption or loss of elastic lamina in the wall of aneurysm.

Mycotic/infectious/septic aneurysms show evidence of significant inflammation/infection in the wall and are often associated with infective endocarditis. The most common organisms include *Staphylococcus aureus*, *Streptococcus viridans* and *Aspergillus sp. Fusiform aneurysms and dolichoectasia* (elongated, wide and tortuous vessel more than 4.5 mm in diameter) arise from the mid-portions rather than the branching points of an artery and are common in the vertebro-basilar circulation. They are seen in patients with advanced atherosclerosis. *Dissecting aneurysm* is dissection (extravasation of blood into the arterial wall through an intimal tear, usually between media and intima) associated with focal arterial dilatation.

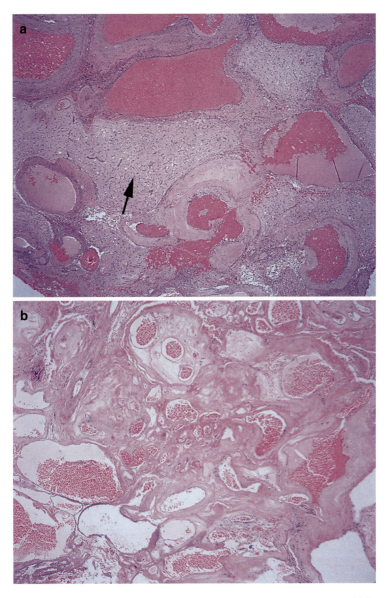

Fig. 4.10 (**a**) Arterio-venous malformation showing thick- and thin-walled vessels with intervening brain tissue (*arrow*), (**b**) cavernous angioma containing closely apposed hyalinised blood vessels. H&E stain

They are common in the vertebro-basilar circulation and can occur with trivial trauma, particularly in patients with an underlying disorder such as Marfan's syndrome, Ehler-Danlos syndrome, polycystic kidney disease and osteogenesis imperfect. Rarely, aneurysms can form in association with neoplasms and several cerebral microangiopathies (Charcot-Bouchard microaneurysm) [10, 11].

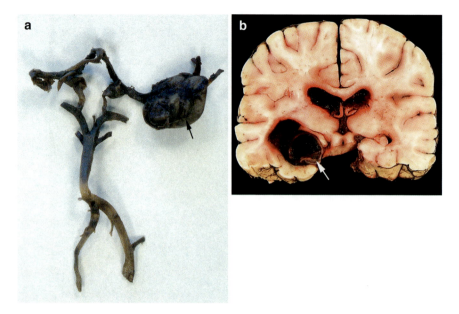

Fig. 4.11 (**a**) Aneurysm arising from the middle cerebral artery (*arrow*), (**b**) ruptured middle cerebral artery aneurysm (*arrow*) with extension of blood into the ventricle

4.3   Consequences of Cerebrovascular Diseases

The various diseases affecting the CNS blood vessels can ultimately lead to two basic types of pathologies, either (1) obstruction of the vessel resulting in ischaemia or infarction, or (2) rupture of the vessel resulting in haemorrhage.

4.3.1   Ischaemia and Infarction

The reduction in cerebral blood flow results in ischaemia and/or infarction. The cerebral ischaemia affects the neurons first as they are the most vulnerable of all the cells, and can be either focal (confined to a defined vascular territory) or global (blood flow to the whole brain is reduced).

The ischaemic infarcts can be classified into the following well-defined groups-(1) large vessel atherosclerotic, (2) small vessel/lacunar, (3) embolic and, (4) crypto-genic. The atherosclerotic plaques within the large arteries can narrow the vascular lumen leading to stagnant blood flow, local thrombosis and occlusion. The extent of infarction depends on the adequacy of collateral circulation. The lacunar stroke (lacunes = small lakes) results from narrowing of deep penetrating arteries due to microatheroma or lipohyalinosis. Diabetes mellitus and hypertension are the two most common predisposing conditions for small vessel disease. Lacunes are seen in basal ganglia, internal capsule, thalamus, corona radiata and brainstem. Embolic

Table 4.6 Morphology of ischaemic injury

Infarct	Macroscopy	Microscopy
Acute (1–4 days)	Mild softening and swelling of the affected area best appreciated by palpation. By 48 h, the area becomes discoloured and well demarcated from the non-infarcted tissue (Fig. 4.12a).	*Few hours- 1 day:* Neuronal eosinophilia (red neurons) with pyknosis, neuropil vacuolation and neutrophil infiltration (Fig. 4.13a, b). *2 days:* Macrophages appear and persist for months (Fig. 4.13c).
Subacute (5–30 days)	Tissue shrinkage and partial cystic changes (Fig. 4.12b).	*5 days:* Astrocytes appear and neutrophils disappear. *Around 1 week:* Astrocytes increase and new blood vessels appear. Numerous macrophages and admixed residual necrotic tissue. Astrocytosis and calcification in adjacent non-infarcted tissue.
Chronic (weeks-months or years)	Extensively cystic and surrounded by atrophic tissue.	Occasional macrophages, haemosiderin pigment (if there is haemorrhage), scattered small blood vessels and fibrillary gliosis in adjacent tissue (Fig. 4.13d).

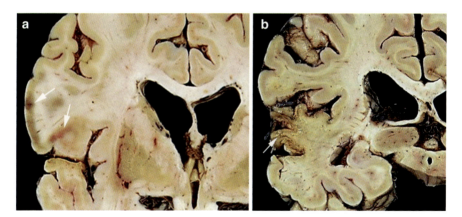

Fig. 4.12 (a) Coronal slice of brain showing focal cortical discolouration and blurring of grey-white matter junction (*arrows*) suggestive of early infarct, (b) an old infarct in the left temporal lobe showing cortical breakdown and yellow-brown discolouration (*arrow*)

strokes usually originate from an embolus within the heart most commonly from an intracardiac thrombi or valvular heart disease. Other uncommon causes for stroke include- arterial dissection, vasculitis, blood disorders, hypotension and tumours. Cryptogenic category is reserved for cases where no definite diagnosis is reached even after extensive investigation.

The morphology of ischaemic injury (Table 4.6) largely depends on duration of the vascular occlusion. If the occlusion is minimal or brief, only vulnerable cells like neurons and oligodendroglia will be affected and the pathological changes may be

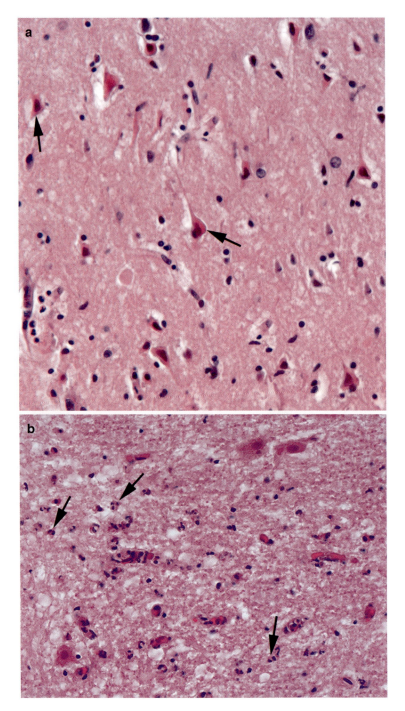

Fig. 4.13 (**a**) Early hypoxic-ischaemic change showing eosinophilic neurons with pyknotic nuclei (*arrows*), (**b**) Early infarct showing infiltration by neutrophil polymorphs (*arrows*), (**c**) Subacute infarct showing foamy macrophages (*right*) and reactive astrocytes (*left*), (**d**) Chronic infarct with cavitation and sparse macrophages (*right*) surrounded by dense gliosis (*left*). H&E stain

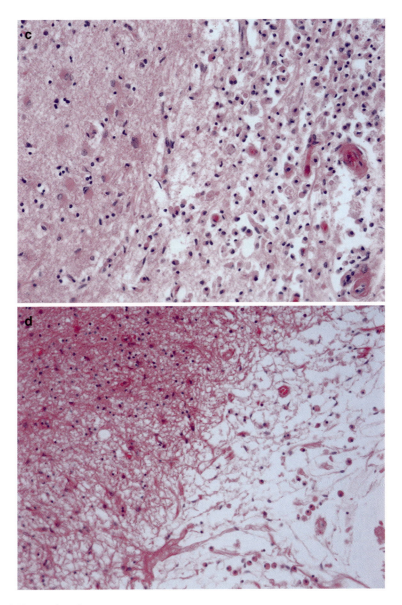

Fig. 4.13 (continued)

temporary. More severe or longer lasting ischaemia result in individual cell necrosis which may elicit a microglial response with little or no infiltrating blood-borne leukocytes. If the insult is severe and prolonged then there will be tissue necrosis, infiltration by blood-borne leukocytes and oedema due to blood-brain barrier breakdown. This tissue necrosis or infarction within a vascular territory is typical of focal brain ischaemia. The necrotic centre in focal brain ischaemia is surrounded by a rim of less severely injured tissue zone termed '*penumbra*' which can be salvaged by appropriate treatment ('therapeutic window').

Global ischaemia results when there is severe reduction in cerebral perfusion pressure either due to severe systemic hypotension (cardiac arrest, dysrhythmia, cardiac tamponade, traumatic haemorrhage) or raised intracranial pressure (commonly severe head injury). There is selective vulnerability of different brain regions to global ischaemia. In adults, the hippocampal CA1 region (Sommer sector), cortical neurons (layers 3 and 5), Purkinje neurons of cerebellum and water-shed or border zone areas are most vulnerable. In infants, the subiculum, basal ganglia, thalamus and brainstem are more vulnerable. The distribution of lesions is similar to those seen in cerebral hypoxia.

Cerebral venous sinus thrombosis (CVT) was once considered a universally fatal disease with diagnosis usually established at autopsy. With the advent of newer imaging modalities (MR angiography, venography) and early recognition, fatal cases are becoming less frequent. It may present with clinical symptoms of benign intracranial hypertension, and non-specific symptoms including headache and seizures. CVT can affect all age groups, but is more common in young women. There are various conditions which predispose to CVT which include pregnancy and puerperium, oral contraceptive use, infections, coagulopathies, dehydration, malignancy, malnutrition, systemic illnesses and autoimmune states. The most common sites of thrombosis are superior sagittal sinus, transverse sinuses and straight sinus. The brain shows bilateral, symmetric areas of haemorrhagic necrosis/infarction and severe oedema. An occluding thrombus is usually identified within one or all of the venous sinuses. Many newer interventional techniques have been developed to dissolve or fragment the clot and have achieved high success rates and good clinical outcomes.

4.3.2   Haemorrhage

Parenchymal/intracerebral haemorrhage is a subtype of stroke with high morbidity and mortality accounting for about 18–48 % of all deaths from stroke [12]. Depending on the underlying cause of bleeding, the haemorrhage can be classified as either primary or secondary (Table 4.7). The primary causes account for approximately 85 % of cases.

The most common sites of haemorrhage are cerebral hemispheres, basal ganglia (Fig. 4.14), thalamus, pons and cerebellum. In the acute stages, the haemorrhage consists of a liquid or semiliquid mass of blood with surrounding oedema. After a few days, the haematoma changes its consistency and adopts a brown colour, while oedema begins to recede. After several months or years, depending on its size, the haematoma becomes a cystic cavity. Small haemorrhages can be reabsorbed almost completely, leaving behind a small linear scar. Microscopically, in the acute stages, extravasated well-preserved red blood cells (RBC) are noted without any inflammation. Subsequently, the RBC begins to lyse and neutrophils appear. This is followed by infiltration of macrophages whose main role is to phagocytose blood products and necrotic tissue. Months to years later a cavity bordered by glial cells, residual macrophages and haemosiderin is all that remains.

Table 4.7 Causes of intracerebral haemorrhage

Primary	Secondary
Chronic hypertension	Trauma
Cerebral amyloid angiopathy (CAA)	Ruptured aneurysm
	Vascular malformations
	Tumours (primary & metastatic)
	Coagulopathies
	Drugs (amphetamines, cocaine) or alcohol
	Haemorrhagic conversion of cerebral infarct
	Vasculitis
	Pregnancy (eclampsia, venous thrombosis)

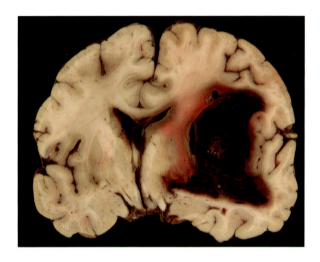

Fig. 4.14 Coronal slice of brain from a case of chronic hypertension showing right basal ganglia haemorrhage with mass effect

Subarachnoid haemorrhage (SAH) refers to collection of blood within the subarachnoid space either alone or in continuity with bleeding elsewhere in the CNS. The most common cause of spontaneous SAH is rupture of aneurysm. The other causes include trauma, vascular malformations, coagulopathies and haematological malignancies. Complications associated with SAH include arterial vasospasm with delayed cerebral ischaemia, raised intracranial pressure and hydrocephalus and rarely hypothalamic infarcts.

Trauma is the most important cause for subdural and extradural haemorrhage which will be discussed in Chap. 13.

References

1. Camejo G, Hurt-Camejo E, Wiklund O, Bondjers G. Association of apo B lipoproteins with arterial proteoglycans: pathological significance and molecular basis. Atherosclerosis. 1998;139(2):205–22.
2. Humphries SE, Morgan L. Genetic risk factors for stroke and carotid atherosclerosis: insights into pathophysiology from candidate gene approaches. Lancet Neurol. 2004;3(4):227–35.

3. Zannad F, Benetos A. Genetics of intima-media thickness. Curr Opin Lipidol. 2003;14(2):191–200.
4. Spangler KM, Challa VR, Moody DM, Bell MA. Arteriolar tortuosity of the white matter in aging and hypertension. A microradiographic study. J Neuropathol Exp Neurol. 1994;53(1):22–6.
5. Nicoll JA, Yamada M, Frackowiak J, Mazur-Kolecka B, Weller RO. Cerebral amyloid angiopathy plays a direct role in the pathogenesis of Alzheimer's disease. Pro-CAA position statement. Neurobiol Aging. 2004;25(5):589–97; discussion 603–4.
6. Joutel A, Favrole P, Labauge P, Chabriat H, Lescoat C, Andreux F, et al. Skin biopsy immunostaining with a Notch3 monoclonal antibody for CADASIL diagnosis. Lancet. 2001;358(9298):2049–51.
7. Maeda A, Yamada M, Itoh Y, Otomo E, Hayakawa M, Miyatake T. Computer-assisted three-dimensional image analysis of cerebral amyloid angiopathy. Stroke. 1993;24(12):1857–64.
8. McCormick WF, Boulter TR. Vascular malformations ("angiomas") of the dura mater. J Neurosurg. 1966;25(3):309–11.
9. Challa VR, Moody DM, Brown WR. Vascular malformations of the central nervous system. J Neuropathol Exp Neurol. 1995;54(5):609–21.
10. Challa VR, Moody DM, Bell MA. The Charcot-Bouchard aneurysm controversy: impact of a new histologic technique. J Neuropathol Exp Neurol. 1992;51(3):264–71.
11. Auerbach ID, Sung SH, Wang Z, Vinters HV. Smooth muscle cells and the pathogenesis of cerebral microvascular disease ("angiomyopathies"). Exp Mol Pathol. 2003;74(2):148–59.
12. Moulin T, Tatu L, Vuillier F, Berger E, Chavot D, Rumbach L. Role of a stroke data bank in evaluating cerebral infarction subtypes: patterns and outcome of 1,776 consecutive patients from the Besancon stroke registry. Cerebrovasc Dis. 2000;10(4):261–71.

Chapter 5
Infections

Abstract The nervous tissue is well protected by the bone, meningeal coverings and an immune system, from invasion by microbes. A breach in the protective barriers or a deficiency of the immune system may result in infection by various microorganisms such as bacteria, viruses, fungi and protozoa. This chapter begins with the list of terms used to describe infections in different neuroanatomical locations. The microorganisms causing CNS infection may be confined to certain geographic locations, affect specific neuroanatomical compartments and specific age groups. This chapter discusses some of the more common infections affecting the CNS worldwide with an emphasis on the role of brain biopsy and other newer microbiological tests in diagnosing these infectious diseases.

Keywords Infection • Microorganisms • Meningitis • Encephalitis • Abscess

The nervous system is protected by the skull and vertebral column, meninges, and blood–brain barrier, from a wide variety of infectious agents. When one or more of these protective barriers are breached, the infectious agents gain access to the CNS tissue and cause infections which have high mortality and morbidity. Infections are caused by bacteria, viruses, fungi, and parasites. The blood-borne route is the most common, but direct invasion and spread along the peripheral nerves can also occur.

Infections can affect different compartments within the nervous system. Some of the commonly used terms to describe the site and nature of an infectious process are listed below, along with their definitions.

Meningitis: Inflammation/infection confined to the leptomeninges with exudate in the subarachnoid space. Spread of infection into the parenchyma may follow. Long-term complications include obstruction of CSF flow resulting in hydrocephalus, and cranial nerve palsies from the thick basal exudate. Viral (lymphocytic) meningitis is more common than bacterial (purulent) meningitis.

Empyema: Collection of pus within the epidural or subdural space. Infection commonly results from local spread or direct contamination (sinusitis, otitis media, trauma or neurosurgery).

Abscess: Accumulation of pus and necrotic tissue within the parenchyma which is generally walled off by fibrovascular capsule and gliosis.

© Springer International Publishing Switzerland 2015

D.A. Hilton, A.G. Shivane, *Neuropathology Simplified: A Guide for Clinicians and Neuroscientists*, DOI 10.1007/978-3-319-14605-8_5

Cerebritis: A purulent non-encapsulated parenchymal infection, which is a stage before abscess formation, where the cerebral parenchyma is infiltrated by acute inflammatory cells.

Encephalitis: Inflammation/infection of the brain usually secondary to a viral infection. There will be necrosis, perivascular lymphocyte cuffing, microglial nodules, viral inclusions and gliosis.

Myelitis: Inflammation/infection of spinal cord parenchyma.

Radiculitis/neuritis: Inflammation/infection of nerve roots.

5.1 Bacterial Infections

5.1.1 Acute Bacterial Meningitis

This is the most common pyogenic infection of the CNS and carries high morbidity and mortality. The causative bacteria are different in different age groups (Table 5.1). The incidence of *Haemophilus influenzae type b* meningitis has reduced drastically in nations which have introduced the conjugate vaccine. Infection most commonly occurs through the haematogenous route, but can also complicate trauma, neurosurgical operations and spread through contiguous foci of infection. Bacteria incite an inflammatory reaction by recruiting polymorphonuclear leucocytes/neutrophils to the site of infection, which then release an array of cytokines and chemokines which result in tissue injury.

The typical CSF findings in bacterial meningitis include marked pleiocytosis, containing predominantly neutrophils, raised protein and reduced glucose. Gram staining may be useful in identifying bacteria. Macroscopic examination of the brain may reveal a purulent exudate in the subarachnoid space over the cerebral convexity (Fig. 5.1a). The exudate may be scanty in patients dying acutely or in those treated with antibiotics. The brain is usually swollen and oedematous. The ventricles may be compressed due to oedema or dilated due to obstruction. Histology shows large numbers of neutrophils within the subarachnoid space (Fig. 5.1b, c) and also along perivascular Virchow-Robin spaces. Intra- or

Table 5.1 Aetiology of bacterial meningitis

Age	Common organisms
Neonate (<1 month)	*Escherichia coli, Klebsiella sp., Citrobacter sp., Listeria monocytogenes, Staphylococcus epidermidis, Staphylococcus aureus.*
Children (1 month- 16 years)	*Haemophilus influenzae type b, Neisseria meningitidis (Meningococcus), Streptococcus agalactiae (Group B β-haemolytic Streptococci), Streptococcus pneumoniae (Pneumococcus).*
Adults & elderly	*Streptococcus pneumoniae (Pneumococcus), Neisseria meningitidis (Meningococcus), Gram-negative bacilli (Escherichia coli, Klebsiella sp., Pseudomonas sp.), Listeria monocytogenes.*

extracellular bacteria may be identified with a Gram stain (Fig. 5.1d). With time, the neutrophils are replaced by chronic inflammatory cells and the exudate transforms into fibrous tissue. The inflammatory cells also invade blood vessels resulting in thrombosis and focal infarcts. Invasion of the ventricular wall results in purulent ventriculitis. The complications of acute bacterial meningitis include-cerebral infarction, obstructive or communicating hydrocephalus, subdural hygroma and subdural empyema.

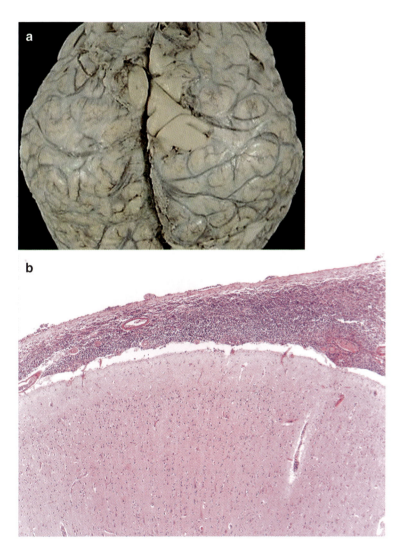

Fig. 5.1 (**a**) Brain showing yellowish exudate in the leptomeninges, (**b, c**) showing dense infiltrate of neutrophils in the subarachnoid space and relatively unaffected cerebral cortex. H&E stain, (**d**) Gram stain showing positive cocci in pairs and small clusters (*arrows*)

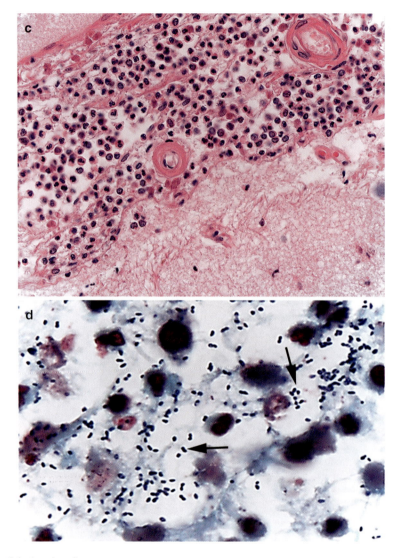

Fig. 5.1 (continued)

5.1.2 Abscess

Epidural abscess is a collection of purulent exudate outside the dura mater. This is more common in the spine than the intracranial compartment. The infection is usually secondary to vertebral osteomyelitis, trauma, surgery or sinusitis. It extends along several vertebral levels. The intracranial epidural abscess appears bi-convex in shape and is bordered by skull and dura mater. Histology reveals neutrophils within the purulent exudate and granulation tissue.

Subdural abscess or empyema is a collection of purulent exudate underneath the dura mater and outside the leptomeninges. The infection does not cross the midline. The infection commonly results from local spread (sinusitis, otitis media, and osteomyelitis), trauma, and neurosurgery. Spread from adjacent purulent leptomeningitis may result in subdural empyema in infants. They can be difficult to diagnose on CT scan and therefore, contrast enhanced MRI scan is preferred.

Intraparenchymal/Brain abscess is the most frequent space-occupying infection and commonly occurs due to spread from a local septic focus (like sinusitis, otitis media, and tooth infection) or blood-borne (bacterial endocarditis, bronchiectasis). The various bacteria isolated from a brain abscess include- *Streptococcus milleri*, *staphylococci*, *Bacteroides sp.*, *Actinomyces sp.*, and gram-negative bacilli. Risk factors include trauma, neurosurgery and immunodeficiency states. Abscesses resulting from local septic focus are commonly localised to frontal/temporal lobes or cerebellum whereas those resulting from haematogenous spread are localised to the junction between grey and white matter and can be multiple. In the earlier stages, the gross examination of the brain may show only focal congestion surrounded by oedema. This will then progress to a well delineated abscess with outer capsule and necrotic centre (Fig. 5.2). Histologically, the evolution of an abscess can be divided into the following stages- focal cerebritis (days 1–3), late cerebritis (days 4–9), early abscess capsule (days 10–13) and well-formed abscess with firm capsule (from day 14). A well-formed abscess has the following four layers- central necrosis, granulation tissue infiltrated by acute and chronic inflammatory cells, fibrous capsule and reactive brain tissue with gliosis. Serious complications of brain abscess include raised intracranial pressure/herniation and purulent ventriculitis.

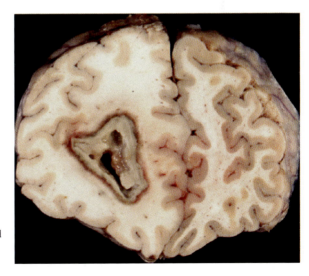

Fig. 5.2 Coronal slice of anterior frontal lobe showing an abscess filled with pus and surrounded by hyperaemia and oedema

5.1.3   Chronic Bacterial Infections

Tuberculosis (TB) caused by *Mycobacterium tuberculosis* can involve different compartments within the CNS and can present as epidural/subdural or parenchymal abscesses, tuberculous meningitis and tuberculomas.

Tuberculous meningitis (TBM) is the most common form of CNS TB which occurs either through haematogenous spread from a primary (usually pulmonary) infection or reactivation of latent infection elsewhere in the body. TBM is more common in developing nations, particularly Asia and Africa. In TBM, a thick exudate accumulates over the base of the brain covering the basal cisterns, brainstem and rarely the spinal cord. In advanced infection, the exudate may extend to involve the cerebral convexities also. With time, the basal exudate becomes more fibrous and cause CSF obstruction resulting in hydrocephalus or cranial nerve palsies. The CSF analysis reveals pleiocytosis containing predominantly lymphocytes, raised protein and reduced glucose. Histologically, there is a dense infiltrate of chronic inflammatory cells composed of lymphocytes, plasma cells, epithelioid macrophages and multinucleated giant cells forming granulomas. The granulomas or tubercles may contain central area of necrosis. Ziehl-Neelsen stain may show variable numbers of acid-fast bacilli (Fig. 5.3). The inflammation can also affect the arterial walls (endarteritis obliterans) resulting in ischaemic complications. Confirmation is either by culture (which takes around 6–8 weeks) or polymerase chain reaction (PCR) testing based on amplification of rRNA derived from *M. tuberculosis* (takes approximately 6–8 h) [1, 2].

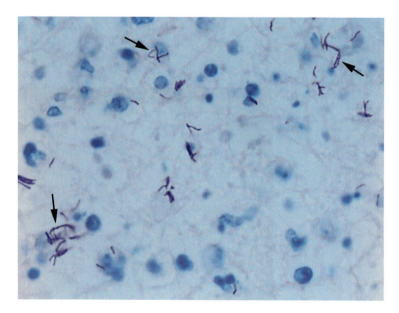

Fig. 5.3 Ziehl-Neelsen stain showing numerous acid fast bacilli (*arrows*) in a case of CNS tuberculosis

Tuberculomas are rounded or multilobular lesions containing a central area of caseous necrosis surrounded by granulomatous reaction composed of lymphocytes, occasional plasma cells, epithelioid macrophages, multinucleated giant cells and variable fibrosis. Tubercle bacilli can be difficult to detect in these lesions. Tuberculomas present clinically as mass lesions and can become cystic, calcified or rupture into the meninges causing meningitis.

TB of the spine (Pott's disease) which involves the vertebral bodies and intervertebral discs commonly results in epidural or subdural abscess. Parenchymal tubercular abscesses have been reported in immunosuppressed and AIDS patients and are histologically similar to pyogenic abscess. The granulomatous reaction is less prominent as a result of reduced cell-mediated immunity and numerous tubercle bacilli are present in the necrotic pus. Infections by non-tuberculous mycobacteria also termed 'atypical mycobacteria' (*Mycobacterium avium-intracellulare complex, M. fortuitum, M. kansasii*) are one of the common causes of opportunistic infection in patients with AIDS.

Syphilis is caused by the spirochete *Treponema pallidum* and presents initially as a chancre at the site of inoculation (primary syphilis). The spirochetes then disseminate through blood and manifests as lymphadenopathy, rash, or mucous patches (secondary syphilis). Patients may then progress to latent stage (latent syphilis) which may last for months or years, or develop cardiovascular, ocular, neuroparenchymal and gummatous lesions (tertiary syphilis). Maternal infection can give rise to congenital neurosyphilis in the foetus. The discovery of penicillin saw a dramatic reduction in syphilis cases, but the disease is re-emerging since the advent of HIV infection.

CNS lesions can manifest within a few years after the initial infection as syphilitic meningitis, meningovascular syphilis, or after the latency of decades as parenchymatous (general paresis of the insane and tabes dorsalis) and gummatous neurosyphilis. *Syphilitic meningitis* is a chronic meningitis composed of lymphocytes and plasma cells. In *meningovascular syphilis* the inflammation involves arteries (Heubner arteritis) and result in ischaemic lesions in the brain or spinal cord. *General paresis of the insane* presents with cognitive and motor disturbances and leads to death. The brain appears atrophic and firm with opaque leptomeninges. Microscopic examination shows cortical neuronal loss, gliosis and proliferation of microglia (rod cells). The spirochetes may occasionally be demonstrated using silver stain. *Tabes dorsalis* is due to degeneration of posterior columns secondary to chronic inflammation within the dorsal nerve roots and dorsal root ganglia. The spirochetes are absent in these lesions. A gumma is a round, firm, rubbery lesion with central necrosis and surrounded by a granulomatous reaction, similar to those seen in tuberculomas.

Borreliosis is a spirochetal infection transmitted by tick and louse bites and includes relapsing fever (*Borrelia recurrentis and other Borrelia* sp.) and Lyme disease (*Borrelia burgdorferi*). Lyme disease is a multisystem disorder common in northern temperate regions and involves the skin, cardiovascular system, joints, and peripheral and central nervous systems. The typical initial skin lesion which appears as maculopapular rash is referred to as 'erythema chronicum migrans'. The nervous system lesions include chronic meningitis, parenchymal chronic inflammatory infiltrates, cranial nerve palsies (commonly facial nerve), and polyradiculitis. Late complications include axonal neuropathies and encephalopathy.

Leptospirosis is caused by the spirochetes of the genus *Leptospira*. The infection is transmitted by water contaminated with rat's urine. CNS lesions include lymphocytic meningitis, subarachnoid and intracerebral haemorrhage and occasionally encephalitis or myelitis.

Brucellosis (*Malta fever*) is caused by aerobic Gram-negative bacteria *Brucella* sp., which is transmitted by raw dairy products and by direct contact with animal products such as the placenta. Neurobrucellosis can manifest as diffuse chronic meningitis, encephalomyelitis, radiculitis and neuritis (particularly acoustic nerves) and vasculitis.

Actinomycosis is caused by anaerobic, filamentous, Gram-positive bacteria, *Actinomyces israeli* and *Actinomyces bovis*. They are commonly found in the oral cavity or in the large intestine as commensals and enter tissues through breaks in the mucosa. CNS lesions are uncommon and occur through either direct extension or via the bloodstream from a focus elsewhere in the body. In brain, they present as multilocular abscesses with central necrosis, acute or chronic inflammatory cells, granulation tissue and filamentous bacteria forming yellowish-brown sulphur granules. Other lesions include meningitis, meningoencephalitis, subdural empyema and epidural abscess.

Nocardiosis is caused mainly by *Nocardia asteroides*, a ubiquitous filamentous aerobic organism. They cause brain abscess or meningitis in debilitated or immunosuppressed patients. Haematogenous spread from a primary pulmonary infection is the commonest route. The spinal cord may be occasionally affected. The abscesses contain thick fibrous walls and acute inflammatory exudate. The organism can be identified using Grocott's silver stain.

Whipple's disease is a multisystem disorder first described by George H. Whipple in 1907, later discovered to be caused by a Gram-positive actinomycete *Tropheryma whippleii*. The disease is common in men between fourth and seventh decades and predominantly involves the intestinal tract. The neurological disease develops in a minority of patients and includes dementia, ophthalmoplegia, hypothalmo-pituitary dysfunction and myoclonus. The lesions are present throughout the CNS and microscopically show accumulation of bacteria-laden macrophages around blood vessels, variable lympho-plasmacytic response, and gliosis. The bacteria are PAS-, Gram- and methanamine silver positive and appear as sickle-shaped inclusions within the macrophages or extracellular tissue. The diagnosis can readily be made by small intestinal biopsy or by PCR testing for specific bacterial 16S rRNA [3].

Rickettsia and Mycoplasma infections of the CNS are relatively rare. Rickettsiae have staining characteristics similar to Gram-negative coccobacilli and cause typhus group infections, spotted fever and Q fever. They are transmitted by ticks or mites, fleas, or lice. Rickettsiae organisms cause damage to blood vessels. The brain in fatal cases may show oedema, perivascular lymphocytes and macrophages, micro-infarcts, or haemorrhages. Mycoplasma are organisms which lack cell wall. *Mycoplasma pneumoniae* cause pneumonia in children and young adults.

Neurological complications are seen in less than 5 % of cases and include meningitis, encephalomyelitis, cerebral infarction, and polyradiculitis. Diagnosis is usually confirmed by serology and PCR testing.

5.2 Viral Infections

5.2.1 Aseptic Meningitis

Aseptic meningitis can be caused by a wide range of viruses (*echovirus, coxsackie virus, herpes simplex virus 2, mumps virus, HIV, lymphochoriomeningitis virus, arboviruses, measles virus, parainfluenza virus, adenovirus*), non-viral infections (e.g. partially-treated bacterial meningitis, syphilis), inflammatory diseases (e.g. Behcet's disease), tumours (e.g. dermoid and epidermoid cysts) and adverse reaction to drugs (e.g. ibuprofen, antibiotics). The CSF analysis reveals pleiocytosis containing predominantly lymphocytes, mildly raised protein and usually a normal glucose. This is usually a benign self-limited condition characterised by a scanty infiltrate of chronic inflammatory cells within the leptomeninges, around superficial cortical vessels and choroid plexus.

5.2.2 Encephalitis or Encephalomyelitis

Viral encephalitis or encephalomyelitis can be acute, subacute or chronic. CNS infection is secondary to active infection elsewhere in the body or more commonly reactivation of dormant infection. Certain basic neuropathological features common to all viral encephalitides include (1) neuronal destruction and engulfment by macrophages (neuronophagia), (2) perivascular chronic inflammatory cells, (3) microglial nodules, and (4) intranuclear or intracytoplasmic viral inclusions. Some of the common viral infections affecting the CNS are described in more detail below.

Poliomyelitis (polio=grey matter) is caused by poliovirus, an enterovirus, and rarely by other enteroviruses and arboviruses. The virus infects the anterior horn cells of the spinal cord. The neurons within the brain may also be affected (*polioencephalitis*). The incidence of poliomyelitis has markedly declined since the introduction of polio vaccine, but occasional outbreaks still occur in developing countries. In the acute phase, the spinal grey matter shows mixed inflammation, anterior horn cell destruction and microglial reaction. The neurons in the brain stem, cerebellum and motor cortex may also be involved. In long-term survivors of poliomyelitis there is marked depletion of anterior horn cells from the spinal cord, scant inflammation, atrophy and grey discolouration of anterior spinal nerve roots and wasting of involved muscles. A syndrome of increasing muscle weakness and atrophy which develops years after the initial infection is referred to as *post-polio syndrome* [4, 5].

Herpes simplex virus (*HSV*) *encephalitis* is the commonest cause of acute encephalitis. Two types of herpes simplex viruses (HSV1 and HSV2) infect the CNS. The infection in adults is mainly caused by HSV1 whereas HSV2 infects the neonates and immunocompromised individuals. Initial primary infection (oropharyngeal in HSV1, genital in HSV2) is followed by latency in the sensory ganglia. Reactivation of the virus results in recurrent mucocutaneous lesions and CNS involvement. Various hypotheses have been postulated for the spread of virus into the CNS- (1) spread along the olfactory nerve fibers and tracts, (2) spread of reactivated virus from trigeminal ganglia, and (3) reactivation of latent infection within the temporal lobes and other regions generally affected in HSV encephalitis. Patients dying in the acute stage show brain swelling, asymmetric haemorrhagic and necrotic lesions within the temporal lobe, cingulate gyrus, orbitofrontal region and insular cortex (limbic regions) (Fig. 5.4a). Microscopic lesions in acute infection include scanty chronic inflammation within the leptomeninges, grey and white matter. The neurons may contain eosinophilic inclusions which are best demonstrated with immunohistochemistry using HSV antibodies and also by electron microscopy (Fig. 5.4b). In more advanced stages, there is haemorrhagic necrosis, intense chronic inflammation, neuronophagia and microglial nodules. Inclusions are sparse at this stage. In chronic stages, the affected brain regions become atrophic with cavitation and yellow-brown discolouration. No viral inclusions are identified in chronic stage. *In situ* hybridisation and PCR testing for viral DNA can be utilised to confirm infection.

The herpes simplex virus (HSV1 and HSV2) infection can also involve the spinal cord (*necrotising myelopathy*). The pathologic features are identical to those seen in established encephalitis. An *atypical form* of HSV encephalitis has been recognised where the disease takes a more prolonged course affecting mainly the brainstem. Rarely, the inflammation may be predominantly *granulomatous* (usually in children) mimicking other chronic granulomatous diseases. The *neonatal herpes virus encephalitis* is mainly caused by HSV2. The lesions involve the brain diffusely without any predilection for specific brain regions as seen in adult cases. Viral intranuclear inclusions are abundant and easily recognised. Early treatment with antiviral drugs like acyclovir has reduced the morbidity and mortality from HSV infections significantly.

Varicella-Zoster virus (*VZV*) causes chickenpox (primary infection) and shingles (re-activation of latent infection). CNS may be involved during the primary infection or re-activation of latent infection and the manifestations are cerebellitis, meningoencephalitis, Reye syndrome, myeloradiculitis, vasculopathy and vasculitis. Histologically, there is a necrotising chronic inflammation composed of lymphocytes and macrophages. Viral intranuclear inclusions may be seen. The small or large-sized blood vessels may be affected by a necrotising inflammatory process (vasculitis) causing infarcts or haemorrhages. Several atypical patterns (multifocal lesions, white matter involvement, ventriculitis, brainstem and visual pathway involvement) of infection have been documented in immunosuppressed patients, particularly AIDS patients. VZV infection can also affect foetus and neonates complicated by limb hypoplasia, various CNS and ocular defects and skin lesions.

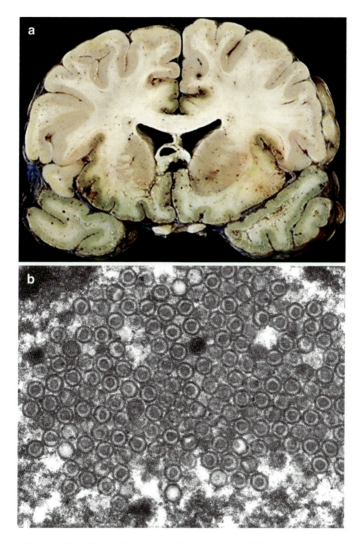

Fig. 5.4 (**a**) Coronal slice of brain from a case of herpes encephalitis showing haemorrhagic areas within both temporal lobes, insulae and cingulate cortices. Note green discolouration due to incidental jaundice. (**b**) Ultrastructural examination showing rounded viral particles from a case of neonatal herpes virus hepatitis

Epstein-Barr virus causes infectious mononucleosis and is also associated with lymphoproliferative disorders and other neoplasms (nasopharyngeal, poorly differentiated or lymphoepithelioma-like carcinomas) [6]. CNS involvement is rare and includes aseptic meningitis, acute disseminated encephalomyelitis, cerebellitis, mono- or polyneuritis, and Guillain-Barre syndrome.

Cytomegalovirus (*CMV*) causes infectious mononucleosis-like syndrome in immunocompetent children and adults. CMV encephalitis and myeloradiculitis are commonly seen in AIDS patients and transplant recipients. The pathology shows variable low-grade or florid, necrotising or non-necrotising encephalitis, ventriculitis and meningomyeloradiculitis with infiltration by lymphocytes and macrophages, microglial nodules and characteristic cytomegalic inclusion cells. The inclusions can be intranuclear or intracytoplasmic and involve neurons, glial cells, endothelial cells and macrophages. The infected cells can be readily identified with immunohistochemistry, *in situ* hybridisation or electron microscopy. Congenital CMV infection is the commonest intra-uterine viral infection. Those who survive the acute illness develop microcephaly, microgyria, porencephalic cysts, hydrocephalus and periventricular calcification.

Rabies, caused by a *rhabdovirus*, is usually transmitted by the bite of a rabid animal. The disease is endemic in Americas, large parts of Europe, Africa and Central Asia. Dogs serve as the main source of human infection but other animal reservoirs include foxes, skunks, raccoons, wolves, jackals, mongoose and bats. There are clinically two distinct forms- the commoner *'furious'* rabies and *'dumb' or 'paralytic'* rabies. The disease is almost always fatal. Neuropathologic examination shows widespread polioencephalomyelitis with microglial nodules (*Babes nodules*) and characteristic eosinophilic rounded cytoplasmic neuronal inclusions termed *'Negri bodies'*. The inclusions are easily recognised in Purkinje neurons of cerebellum and pyramidal hippocampal neurons.

Arboviruses or arthropod-borne viruses are transmitted by bites of insects (mosquito or tick). They belong to four virus families- Togaviridae, Flaviviridae, Bunyaviridae, and Reoviridae. Most of these viruses cause only a mild febrile illness and only a few causes encephalitis. The encephalitides caused by arboviruses have a distinct geographic distribution. Some of the well-known arbovirus encephalitides are listed in Table 5.2.

The Eastern equine and Japanese encephalitis carry high morbidity and mortality. The brain may appear congested and swollen. The neuropathologic examination shows meningeal, perivascular and parenchymal chronic inflammation, neuronophagia and necrosis. Viral inclusions are not seen and confirmation of viral aetiology is by serologic tests, electron microscopy or viral culture.

Rubella virus causes German measles and progressive encephalitis, a delayed complication of congenital or childhood infection. Congenital infection results in teratogenic damage to foetus. The brain abnormalities include microcephaly, hydrocephalus, white matter cavitation, meningoencephalitis and, in chronic stages, mineralisation of basal ganglia. The pathogenesis is presumed to be an autoimmune process. No viral inclusions are identified.

Measles virus, a paramyxovirus, causes aseptic meningitis or acute disseminated encephalomyelitis (ADEM) and also less commonly two subacute or chronic forms of encephalitis- Measles inclusion-body encephalitis and subacute sclerosing panencephalitis (SSPE). Measles inclusion-body encephalitis develops in immunosuppressed patients several months after the initial infection and is usually fatal. Neuropathology reveals areas of chronic inflammation, necrosis and characteristic eosinophilic nuclear inclusions within the neurons and glia. The virus can be detected by immunohistochemistry or electron microscopy. SSPE is a chronic progressive encephalitis which occurs several years after the initial infection. Measles vaccination reduces the risk of SSPE by 10–20 folds [7]. The brain may

Table 5.2 The arbovirus encephalitides

Encephalitides	Geographic distribution	Anatomical regions involved
Eastern equine encephalitis	Eastern parts of USA, Caribbean and South America	Basal ganglia, thalamus, brainstem
Western equine encephalitis	Western parts of USA	Basal ganglia, thalamus, brainstem
Venezuelan equine encephalitis	South and Central America, Florida, South-West USA	Basal ganglia, thalamus, brainstem
St Louis encephalitis	USA, Central & South America	Midbrain, thalamus
Japanese encephalitis	South East Asia, Bangladesh, Pakistan	Thalamus, substantia nigra, brainstem and spinal cord
West Nile fever	Africa, East Europe, West Asia, Middle East	Thalamus, cerebellum, substantia nigra, brainstem and spinal cord
Murray valley encephalitis	South West Australia, New Guinea	Any brain region
Central European encephalitis	Central Europe	Cerebral cortex, basal ganglia, cerebellum, brainstem and spinal cord
Russian spring-summer encephalitis	Russia, East Asia	Cerebral cortex, basal ganglia, cerebellum, brainstem and spinal cord

appear atrophic with abnormally firm and grey discoloured white matter. The histology shows chronic encephalitis, gliosis (Fig. 5.5a, b), Alzheimer's type neurofibrillary tangles (in long-standing cases) [8] and intranuclear eosinophilic inclusions.

Progressive multifocal leukoencephalopathy (PML) is an opportunistic infection, seen in immunosuppressed and AIDS patients and caused by a *Polyoma* virus, JC virus. The virus specifically targets oligodendrocytes resulting in large areas of demyelination involving the posterior hemispheric white matter, cerebral cortex, deep grey nuclei and sometimes also hindbrain and spinal cord. Macroscopically, the lesions appear as asymmetric grey-discoloured necrotic areas within the white matter (Fig. 5.6). The viral particles enlarge oligodendroglial nuclei and appear as pale inclusions. These can be detected by immunohistochemistry (using an antibody to SV40), *in situ* hybridisation or electron microscopy. In more advanced lesions, enlarged or giant astrocytes with bizarre hyperchromatic nuclei can be identified within the demyelinated zones. There is sparse chronic inflammatory cell infiltrate. The disease progresses and eventually results in death. The treatment is aimed at reducing the immunosuppression.

Human immunodeficiency virus (HIV) is a retrovirus of the *Lentivirus* subfamily. The clinical syndrome associated with HIV infection and defined by low CD4-positive T cells (<200/μL) and one of 23 specific illnesses is termed 'Acquired Immunodeficiency Syndrome/AIDS' [9]. The neurological complications of HIV infection include- direct infection of the CNS by the virus (HIV encephalitis, HIV leukoencephalopathy, and diffuse poliodystrophy), various opportunistic infections, neoplasms (mainly lymphomas), changes secondary to systemic HIV

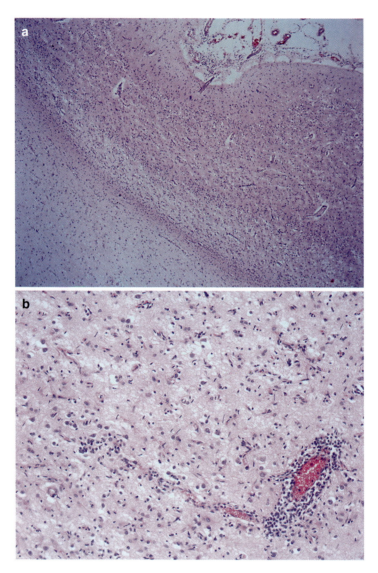

Fig. 5.5 A case of subacute sclerosing panencephalitis showing cerebral cortical atrophy, gliosis (**a**), and chronic perivascular inflammation including prominent microglial cells (**b**). H&E stain

infection, and treatment-related toxicity. *HIV encephalitis* is characterised by a low-grade chronic inflammation, multinucleated giant cells (HIV giant cells), astrocytic and microglial activation (also referred to as 'microglial nodule encephalitis'). The virus is detected within giant cells and microglia by immunohistochemistry (using antibody to HIV gp41 or p24) or *in situ* hybridisation. Any brain region can be affected, but the deep white matter and basal ganglia are frequently involved. *HIV leukoencephalopathy* is characterised by diffuse white matter myelin pallor,

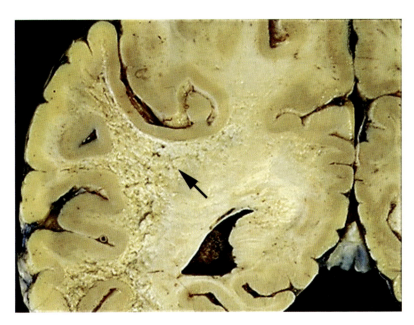

Fig. 5.6 Coronal slice of brain from a case of PML showing grey discoloured, granular area within the white matter (*arrow*)

Table 5.3 Opportunistic infections and neoplasms in HIV/AIDS

Opportunistic infections	Neoplasms
Fungal (*Cryptococcus sp., Aspergillus sp., Coccidioides sp., Histoplasma sp., Candida sp., Mucor sp.*)	Primary CNS lymphoma (EBV-associated)
Virus (*CMV, VZV, HSV, JC virus, Adenovirus, Measles*)	Systemic non-Hodgkin's lymphoma with CNS spread
Parasites (*Toxoplasma*)	
Bacteria (*Mycobacterium avium-intracellulare, M. tuberculosis, Treponema pallidum*)	

axonal loss and gliosis. This is usually associated with HIV encephalitis. Involvement of grey matter resulting in neuronal loss, gliosis and microglial activation is termed 'poliodystrophy'. The neuronal dysfunction results in a dementing illness with memory and personality changes termed '*HIV-associated dementia*' or '*AIDS-dementia complex*'. The spinal cord may also be affected in HIV infection and results in *vacuolar myelopathy*. The pathology resembles subacute combined degeneration of the spinal cord and shows vacuolation of posterior columns and lateral corticospinal tracts, with accumulation of macrophages. Patients treated with anti-retroviral drugs very rarely develop a severe *necrotising leukoencephalopathy*. Children with HIV/AIDS develop progressive encephalitis with prominent areas of dystrophic calcification. Table 5.3 lists the various opportunistic infections and neoplasms in HIV/AIDS.

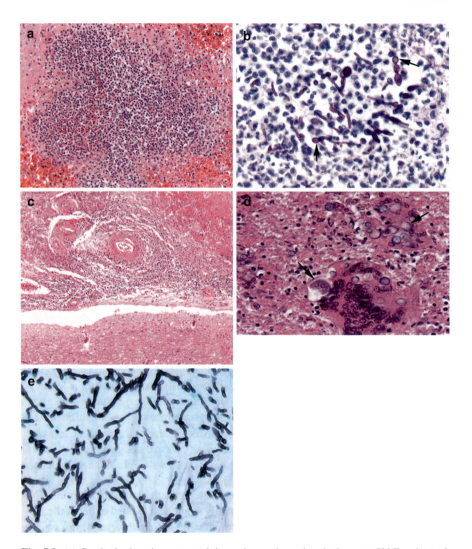

Fig. 5.8 (**a**) Cerebral microabscess containing polymorphonuclear leukocytes (H&E stain) and, (**b**) budding yeasts and pseudo hyphae of *Candida* organisms (*arrows*, PAS stain), (**c**) showing chronic meningitis and, (**d**) multinucleated giant cells containing *Coccidioides* organisms (*arrows*) (H&E stain), (**e**) branching hyphae from a case of *Aspergillus* infection (Grocott stain)

shows perivascular 'ring' haemorrhages within the white matter and focal collections of microglia/macrophages and astrocytes (Durck granuloma). The parasites can be recognised within the red blood cells along with granules of dark malarial pigment.

Toxoplasmosis is caused by a coccidian *Toxoplasma gondii*. Domestic cats serve as definitive hosts and human infection occurs through consumption of undercooked meat or faeces containing parasitic cysts. CNS infection becomes symptomatic when the cell-mediated immunity is reduced. The human infection can occur con-

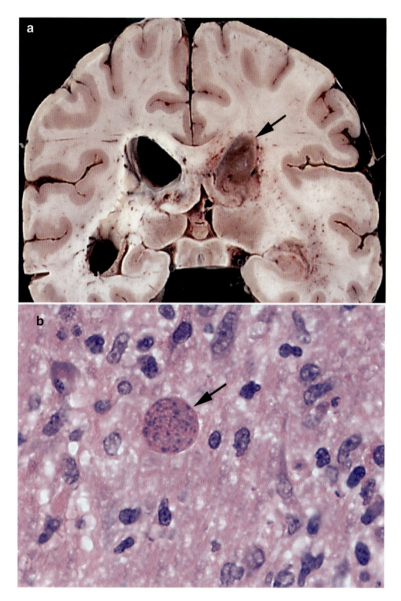

Fig. 5.9 Toxoplasmosis (**a**) Coronal slice of brain showing a haemorrhagic necrotic lesion in the right lateral ventricle (*arrow*), (**b**) Toxoplasma cyst/bradyzoite (*arrow*). H&E stain

genitally (triad of hydrocephalus, cerebral calcification and chorioretinitis) or in adult immunosuppressed individuals (single or multiple ring enhancing necrotising abscesses) (Fig. 5.9a). Any part of the brain may be involved, but basal ganglia and periventricular regions are the most commonly affected areas. Histology shows necrosis and dense infiltration by mainly lymphocytes, and macrophages/microglia.

Table 5.5 Major helminthic infections of the CNS

Cestodes	Trematodes	Nematodes
Cysticercus cellulosae (*larva of Taenia solium*) (Neuro cysticercosis)	*Schistosoma sp.* (Schistosomiasis)	*Strongyloides stercoralis* (Strongyloidiasis)
Echinococcus granulosus (Hydatid cyst)	*Paragonimus westermani* (Paragonimiasis)	*Angiostrongylus cantonensis* (Angiostrongyliasis)
Taenia multiceps (Coenurosis)		*Toxocara canis* (Visceral larva migrans)
Spirometra sp. (Sparganosis)		*Trichinella spiralis* (Trichinosis)
		Filariases (*loa-loa, Dracunculus sp., Onchocerca*)

The *Toxoplasma* cysts (containing bradyzoites) (Fig. 5.9b) and intra- or extracellular tachyzoites are recognised by routine H&E stain or by immunohistochemistry using *Toxoplasma* antibody. As the lesion advances, the necrotic material gets resorbed leaving behind a cystic cavity with little inflammation and rare tachyzoites.

Trypanosomiasis is caused by two species depending on the geographic location, *Trypanosoma brucei* (African trypanosomiasis or sleeping sickness) and *Trypanosoma cruzi* (American trypanosomiasis or Chagas' disease). The African disease is transmitted to humans by bite of tsetse fly. There are two subspecies- *T. b. rhodesiense* and *T. b. gambiense*. The African form presents with fulminant or subacute-chronic meningoencephalitis characterised by lymphoplasma cells and macrophage infiltration, microglial nodules, astrocytosis and rare parasites. The American disease is transmitted by reduviid bugs and can cause acute, chronic or re-activated infections. Acute infections are common in infants and children and are asymptomatic. Symptomatic disease presents as encephalitis or myocarditis. Chronic infection in adults leads to damage of autonomic nervous system. Reactivated infection is seen in immunosuppressed patients and presents as necrotising lesions. The parasites can be recognised within astrocytes or macrophages in routine H&E stain, using immunohistochemistry/fluorescence, *in situ* hybridisation or PCR. The treatment of trypanosomiasis with melarsoprol may rarely result in acute haemorrhagic leukoencephalopathy [10].

5.4.2 Metazoal/Helminthic Infections

Helminthic infections are caused by Cestodes, Trematodes (flat worms) or Nematodes (round worms). Humans can be either the definitive or intermediate host for these infections. Table 5.5 lists the major helminths affecting the CNS.

Cysticercosis is caused by the larval form of pig tapeworm (*Taenia solium*) and is the commonest parasitic infection of the CNS. The disease is common in Latin America, India, sub-Saharan Africa, China and some parts of Europe and USA. The infection can be asymptomatic or present more commonly with epilepsy. Man is the intermediate host and develops infection after ingesting eggs of the pig tapeworm. The eggs hatch into larvae which then pierce the intestinal wall and spread to other tissues including the CNS. The cysts can be solitary or numerous, scattered within the meninges, cerebral cortex or ventricles. The viable cyst contains invaginated scolex with four suckers and hooklets (mouth parts). The cyst wall is layered and has outer cuticular, middle cellular and inner reticular layers. The cysts degenerate, become fibrotic and calcify. No tissue reaction is seen around viable cysts but degenerate or dead cyst can sometimes elicit a florid inflammatory reaction in the surrounding tissue.

Echinococcosis/Hydatidosis is caused by the larvae of dog tapeworm (*Echinococcus granulosus*). The disease is common in Mediterranean countries, the Middle-East, Latin America, sheep-rearing countries like Australia, New Zealand, South Africa, some parts of USA and UK (Wales, Shetland islands). Dogs and other canines serve as definitive hosts and sheep is the intermediate host. Man is an accidental host and acquires infection through ingestion of eggs from food contaminated with canine faeces. The larvae travel to other tissues like liver, lungs and rarely the CNS and form enlarging cysts. The cysts are solitary, unilocular, and contain two distinct layers- outer laminated cuticular and inner germinal layers.

Schistosomiasis is caused by three species of the trematode *Schistosoma* (fluke worm) – *S. japonicum* (endemic in Japan, China and SE Asia), *S. mansoni* (South America, Puerto Rico, West Indies, the Middle East, Africa), and *S. haematobium* (Africa, the Middle East). Man is the definitive host and the trematodes live within the abdominal and pelvic venous plexuses and release eggs into the bloodstream. Further development into larvae occurs outside humans within the snail, which serve as intermediate hosts. CNS infection is uncommon and predominantly involves the spinal cord. The affected spinal segment (usually thoracic or lumbo-sacral) may appear swollen with multiple surface nodules (granulomas). The histology shows eggs surrounded by a mild to florid granulomatous reaction. Rarely, brain may also be affected, especially the cerebral or cerebellar cortex and deep grey nuclei.

Trichinosis is caused by the nematode *Trichinella spiralis* through ingestion of undercooked pork containing encysted larvae. Man serves as both intermediate and final hosts. The adult worm resides in the upper intestines and release larvae which then pierce the intestinal wall to enter various tissues. CNS involvement is uncommon. The larvae encyst within skeletal muscle where they remain dormant for years or cause myositis.

Other nematode infections include- *Angiostrongyliasis* which causes meningitis with a prominent eosinophilic infiltrate; *Strongyloidiasis* common in the tropics and causes massive intestinal infection in immunosuppressed individuals; the clinical syndrome of visceral larva migrans caused by infection with *Toxocara sp.*.

5.5 Role of Brain Biopsy in Infectious Diseases

The brain biopsy is considered when all other diagnostic techniques fail to confirm the aetiological agent for the infectious process. Some mycobacterial infections and chronic fungal infections may necessitate brain biopsy for definitive confirmation.

Infections which present as space occupying lesions, mainly in the setting of immunosuppression, can mimic neoplasms and the only way to solve the dilemma is by performing a biopsy. Brain biopsy may also have a role in atypical infections, multifocal or diffuse infective processes. With the advent of newer diagnostic microbiological tools such as rRNA-based amplification and DNA-based PCR tests, the need for brain biopsy is becoming even less. Many of these PCR tests can be performed on CSF and positivity indicates active infection. However, the positive results on brain tissue may not necessarily indicate active infection as some of the viruses (JC, Herpes) can be detected even in normal brains.

References

1. Lin JJ, Harn HJ, Hsu YD, Tsao WL, Lee HS, Lee WH. Rapid diagnosis of tuberculous meningitis by polymerase chain reaction assay of cerebrospinal fluid. J Neurol. 1995;242(3): 147–52.
2. Shankar P, Manjunath N, Mohan KK, Prasad K, Behari M, Shriniwas, et al. Rapid diagnosis of tuberculous meningitis by polymerase chain reaction. Lancet. 1991;337(8732):5–7.
3. Lynch T, Odel J, Fredericks DN, Louis ED, Forman S, Rotterdam H, et al. Polymerase chain reaction-based detection of Tropheryma whippelii in central nervous system Whipple's disease. Ann Neurol. 1997;42(1):120–4.
4. Tjensvoll AB, Gilhus NE. The post-poliomyelitis syndrome–a real complication. A poliomyelitis material from the Haukeland hospital. Tidsskr Nor Laegeforen. 1997;117(4):510–3.
5. Grehl O, Muller-Naendrup C, Jenni W. Postpolio syndrome: retrospective study in a former polio clinic. Praxis (Bern 1994). 1996;85(1–2):14–20.
6. Purtilo DT, Strobach RS, Okano M, Davis JR. Epstein-Barr virus-associated lymphoproliferative disorders. Lab Invest. 1992;67(1):5–23.
7. Farrington CP. Subacute sclerosing panencephalitis in England and Wales: transient effects and risk estimates. Stat Med. 1991;10(11):1733–44.
8. Mandybur TI. The distribution of Alzheimer's neurofibrillary tangles and gliosis in chronic subacute sclerosing panencephalitis. Acta Neuropathol. 1990;80(3):307–10.
9. Centers for Disease Control (CDC). Revision of the CDC surveillance case definition for acquired immunodeficiency syndrome. Council of State and Territorial Epidemiologists; AIDS Program, Center for Infectious Diseases. MMWR Morb Mortal Wkly Rep. 1987;36 Suppl 1:1S–5.
10. Pepin J, Milord F, Khonde AN, Niyonsenga T, Loko L, Mpia B, et al. Risk factors for encephalopathy and mortality during melarsoprol treatment of Trypanosoma brucei gambiense sleeping sickness. Trans R Soc Trop Med Hyg. 1995;89(1):92–7.

Chapter 6
Tumours of Central Nervous System

Abstract Many different types of primary tumour occur within the central nervous system, and it is also an important site for secondary spread of tumours from elsewhere in the body. Tumours are classified using the World Health Organisation system, which also assigns a biological grade indicating the degree of malignancy without treatment. This chapter describes the principles of tumour classification, the key pathological features of the majority of tumour subtypes and highlights the role of genetic findings in predicting biological behaviour and tumour classification.

Keywords Brain tumour • Genetics • Chemosensitivity • Radiosensitivity • WHO grade

Tumours of the central nervous system (CNS) represent around 3 % of all malignancies, but are the second most common type of tumour in children and young adults and population-based studies indicate an overall incidence of intracranial tumours of approximately 21/100,000 per year [1]. For the purposes of this chapter, we have included some tumours that occur within the cranial and spinal cavities that are not derived from CNS tissues, such as tumours of the meninges, pituitary gland and peripheral nerves.

6.1 Classification

Tumour classification is based on the presumed cell of origin and biological grade of malignancy, which is derived from the microscopic appearances. Most neuropathologists use the World Health Organisation classification system for CNS tumours [2] which has a biological grading system from I-IV, with I being very slow growing and unlikely to spread, to IV being rapidly growing and ability to spread extensively within the CNS (spread outside of the CNS is rare for most primary tumours of the CNS). It should be noted that these biological WHO grades relate to the natural behaviour of the tumour without treatment, so that some WHO Grade IV tumours, (e.g. medulloblastomas), can have a prolonged survival with current therapy. In

© Springer International Publishing Switzerland 2015   79
D.A. Hilton, A.G. Shivane, *Neuropathology Simplified: A Guide for Clinicians and Neuroscientists*, DOI 10.1007/978-3-319-14605-8_6

addition, different genetic subtypes of tumours of the same WHO histological type and grade, vary in their prognosis, which is likely to be reflected in future versions of the WHO classification system.

Although tumours from elsewhere in the body may spread to the CNS, approximately two thirds of intracranial tumours are primary, the majority of which are either of astrocytic origin, meningiomas, pituitary tumours or peripheral nerve sheath tumours. The frequency of each type of tumour varies with age and gender, for example gliomas are more common in men and meningiomas more common in women, and certain tumours such as medulloblastomas, ependymomas, pilocytic astrocytomas, craniopharyngiomas and choroid plexus tumours are more common in childhood.

Tumours may present with a variety of neurological symptoms including signs of raised intracranial pressure (sometimes due to hydrocephalus, particularly in the case of posterior fossa tumours), focal neurological deficits and epilepsy. The aetiology of tumours of the CNS is unknown in the vast majority of cases. Recent data suggests an association between long-term mobile phone and some cases of ipsilateral schwannoma, but evidence for an association with other types of tumour is inconclusive [3, 4]. Tumours may occur as a delayed complication of radiotherapy (particularly meningeal tumours and gliomas), Epstein Barr virus infection may cause lymphoma and there are a number of rare inherited genetic syndromes that predispose to neurological tumours (see Table 6.1).

6.2   Sending Specimens to the Laboratory

It is important that specimens are sent to pathologists with adequate clinical information to allow accurate interpretation of the histological appearances (see Box 3.1). Information that a pathologist requires includes age, gender, family history (particularly of tumours), past medical history (including any treatment such as chemotherapy, radiotherapy and dexamethasone, or previous tumours), symptoms (including duration) and imaging findings (including location of tumour and pattern of contrast enhancement). If preoperative embolisation has been used to reduce bleeding during surgery e.g. for meningiomas, the pathologist must be informed as this can cause tumour necrosis and an increased mitotic rate [5], which can be confused with malignant change. In many cases it may be helpful to the neurosurgeon to have a rapid intraoperative diagnosis to confirm that the tissue is diagnostic and/or to give a provisional histological analysis to guide the extent of surgical resection that is appropriate (see Box 3.2). If an intraoperative diagnosis is planned it is important to warn the pathologist in advance so that laboratory staff can be prepared to deal with a specimen promptly. It is important to inform the laboratory if there is any potential that the patient may harbour a category 3 or 4 pathogen, so that additional precautions can be taken to prevent risk of infection to laboratory staff. A system should be agreed with a local laboratory on how intraoperative specimens are sent, but in general, the specimen should be sent immediately to the laboratory fresh, and should not be allowed to dry out in the process as this will hinder interpretation. Rapid intraoperative diagnoses are made by either freezing the tissue and then cutting 'frozen sections' from this onto

Table 6.1 Familial tumour syndromes involving the CNS

Syndrome	Gene, locus	CNS tumours
Neurofibromatosis type 1	*NF1/neurofibromin*, 17q11	Neurofibromas, malignant nerve sheath tumours, astrocytic tumours, especially pilocytic astrocytoma of optic nerve
Neurofibromatosis type 2	*NF2/merlin*, 22q12	Schwannoma, meningioma, ependymoma
Tuberous sclerosis	*TS1*, 9q34 or *TS2*, 16p13	Sub-ependymal giant cell astrocytoma
von Hippel-Lindau disease	*VHL*, 3p25	Haemangioblastoma
Li-Fraumeni syndrome	*TP53*, 17p13	Astrocytic tumours, primitive neuroectodermal tumours, medulloblastoma, choroid plexus tumours
Gorlin syndrome (Naevoid basal cell carcinoma syndrome)	*PTCH*, 9q22	Medulloblastoma
Cowden syndrome	*PTEN*, 10q23	Dysplastic gangliocytoma of the cerebellum (Lhermitte-Duclos disease)
Turcot syndrome	*APC*, 5q21 (and others)	Medulloblastoma, glioblastoma
Melanoma astrocytoma syndrome	*p16*, 9p	Astrocytic tumour
Familial retinoblastoma	*Retinoblastoma gene*, 13q	Retinoblastoma, pineoblastoma
Multiple endocrine neoplasia type 1	*MEN1*, 11q13	Pituitary adenoma
Rhabdoid tumour predisposition syndrome	*INI1*, 22q11	Atypical teratoid/rhabdoid tumours

a glass slide, or by squashing a small sample of tumour onto a glass slide and making a 'smear preparation'. Tissue for 'permanent' histology is placed in formalin and may be sent to the laboratory separately. In an increasing number of cases fresh tissue may also be required to allow more extensive genetic testing to be undertaken on the tumour, so local laboratory advice should be taken on how tumours should be sent.

6.3   Gliomas

6.3.1   Astrocytic Tumours

These are the most common type of primary CNS tumour, histologically show a resemblance to astrocytes, and express glial fibrillary acidic protein. The different subtypes are listed in Table 6.2.

The term 'diffuse astrocytic tumours' is often used to describe diffuse astrocytomas, anaplastic astrocytomas and glioblastomas, as these tumours tend to be highly

Table 6.2 Astrocytic tumours

Subependymal giant cell astrocytoma (WHO Grade I)
Pilocytic astrocytoma (WHO Grade I)
Pilomyxoid astrocytoma (WHO Grade II)
Pleomorphic xanthoastrocytoma (WHO Grade II)
Diffuse astrocytoma (fibrillary, protoplasmic and gemistocytic subtypes) (WHO Grade II)
Anaplastic astrocytoma (WHO Grade III)
Glioblastoma (including giant cell glioblastoma and gliosarcoma) (WHO Grade IV)

infiltrative, so cannot be completely excised surgically. **Diffuse astrocytomas** (Fig. 6.1) can occur anywhere in the CNS, but predominantly within cerebral hemispheres of adults, and although most are slow growing, as is usually not possible to resect them completely, they recur over a number of years. Average survival is around 5–8 years, and in about half of cases, these tumours transform to high grade tumours, either **anaplastic astrocytomas** or **glioblastomas** (Fig. 6.2). Both of these latter types of tumour occur in the same regions as diffuse astrocytomas, but generally in older adults and they show contrast enhancement on imaging. Histologically, these high grade tumours are more cellular than diffuse astocytomas and have frequent mitoses. In addition, glioblastomas have areas of necrosis and show vascular proliferation. Although glioblastomas may arise from lower grade tumours (secondary glioblastomas), the majority occur *de novo* (primary glioblastomas). Average survival for anaplastic astrocytomas is 2–4 years, and for glioblastomas are around 1 year, although this depends on a number of factors including clinical condition (Karnofsky performance scale), age, treatment and genetic changes within the tumour (see below), with around 5 % patients with glioblastomas surviving 2 years. A list of features used to grade diffuse astrocytic tumours is given in Table 6.3.

Gliomatosis cerebri is defined as a diffuse glioma (usually astrocytic, but sometimes oligodendroglial), involving at least three lobes, and often both cerebral hemispheres, brain stem and cerebellum. The extent of tumour can be seen on T2 and FLAIR weighted MRI, and although histological grading on biopsy can be difficult, most behave as WHO Grade III tumours.

Pilocytic astrocytomas are better circumscribed than the types of astrocytic tumour discussed above, only very rarely progress to more malignant tumours, are more common in children and young adults, and show a predilection for certain sites within the CNS (optic nerve, optic chiasm, hypothalamus and cerebellum). Histologically they are characterised by bipolar astrocytic cells forming solid and microcystic areas, Rosenthal fibres (hyaline accumulations of filamentous material), and vascular proliferation (Fig. 6.3). If they occur at a site where a surgical excision is possible, they have an excellent prognosis. Like high grade diffuse astrocytomas, these may show contrast enhancement on imaging. A related tumour, the **pilomyxoid astrocytoma**, most often occurring in the hypothalamic/chiasmic region of young children, has a more mucoid consistency and perivascular arrangement of tumour cells, but has tendency to recur and spread via the CSF.

Pleomorphic xanthoastrocytomas are generally slow growing gliomas, but can occasionally be aggressive, and frequently present with seizures and on imaging

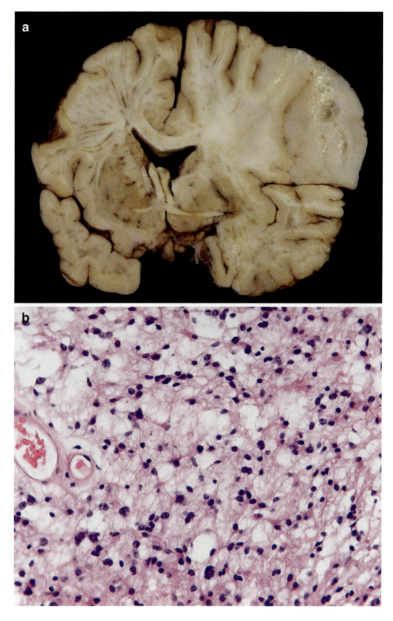

Fig. 6.1 (**a**) Diffuse astrocytoma, showing diffuse expansion of right upper cerebral hemisphere, shift of midline to the left, loss of grey/white matter demarcation and areas of cystic change. (**b**) Histologically is composed of cells with an astrocytic morphology with fairly uniform appearances, low cellularity and absence of mitotic figures. H&E stain

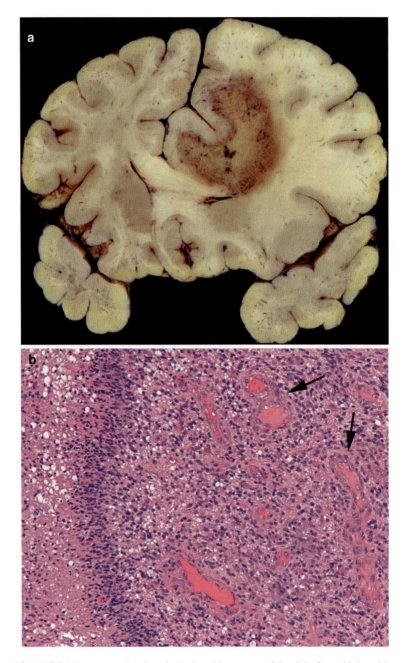

Fig. 6.2 (**a**) Glioblastoma predominantly in the white matter of the right frontal lobe with extensive necrosis (*yellow area*), causing shift of midline structures. (**b**) Microscopically the tumour is composed of astrocytic cells with large irregular nuclei, mitotic figures, area of necrosis (*left*) and vascular proliferation (*arrows*). H&E stain

Table 6.3 Histological features used in grading of diffuse astrocytic tumours

Increased cellularity – WHO Grade II
Nuclear atypia – WHO Grade II
Mitotic activity – WHO Grade III
Vascular proliferation – WHO Grade IV
Tumour necrosis – WHO Grade IV

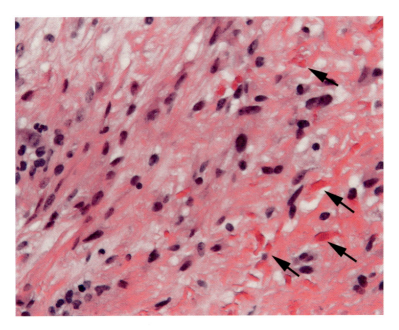

Fig. 6.3 Pilocytic astrocytoma composed of elongate astrocytic cells with irregular eosinophilic proteinaceous droplets (Rosenthal fibres – *arrows*). H&E stain

have a cyst and mural nodule. The tumours often show quite marked cytological atypia and accumulation of cytoplasmic lipid, but usually lack mitotic activity.

Subependymal giant cell astrocytomas occur almost exclusively within the context of tuberous sclerosis and tend to form a predominantly exophytic mass protruding into the ventricles which may cause hydrocephalus. These tumours are composed of pleomorphic and multinucleate astrocytic cells, but are biologically benign.

6.3.2 Genetics of Gliomas

A large number of genetic changes have been described in gliomas, many of which are becoming of diagnostic and clinical relevance and are likely to feature prominently in future World Health Organisation classification systems. Some key genetic changes of clinical relevance are listed in Table 6.4.

Table 6.4 Clinically important genetic changes in gliomas

Genetic change	Comments
Mutations in *isocitrate dehydrogenase* (*IDH*) genes types 1 and 2	Present in about 75 % of diffuse astrocytomas, anaplastic astrocytomas, oligodendrogliomas and anaplastic oligodendrogliomas. Common in secondary glioblastomas.
	Common mutation in *IDH1 gene* (R132H) is responsible for about 90 % all mutations (Fig. 6.4).
	Glioblastomas with *IDH1* mutations have a better prognosis than those without.
Mutations in *alpha-thalassaemia/mental retardation syndrome X-linked* (*ATRX*) gene	Strong association with *IDH* mutations and astrocytic differentiation.
	Present in about 70 % of diffuse astrocytomas and anaplastic astrocytomas.
	Common in secondary glioblastomas.
	Anaplastic astrocytomas with mutation have a better prognosis than those without.
Co-deletion of chromosome arms 1p and 19q	Strong association with *IDH* mutations and oligodendroglial differentiation.
	Present in about 80 % of oligodendrogliomas and anaplastic oligodendrogliomas (Fig. 6.5).
	Predicts high rate of chemosensitivity, radiosensitivity and good prognosis.
Methylation of the *O6-methylguanine-DNA methyl transferase* (*MGMT*) gene promoter	Present in the majority of astrocytic and oligodendrogial tumours.
	Strong association with 1p/19q co-deletion in oligodendrogliomas.
	Predicts chemosensitivity to alkylating agents in glioblastomas.
	Associated with pseudoprogression in glioblastomas.
BRAF gene duplication and fusion	Present in about 60 % of pilocytic astrocytomas.
	Possible target for therapy.
Epidermal growth factor receptor gene rearrangement (*EGFRvIII*)	Found in about 30 % of primary glioblastomas.
	Associated with poor prognosis.
	Possible target for therapy.

6.3.3 Non-astrocytic Gliomas

6.3.3.1 Oligodendrogliomas

These present in a similar way to astrocytic tumours, often with epilepsy, but are very uncommon in childhood. Compared with astrocytic tumours, oligodendrogliomas are more often cortically based, may undergo haemorrhage and often show evidence of calcification on imaging. A key difference with astrocytic tumours is that a high proportion show both chemosensitivity and radiosensitivity. Microscopically they are composed of cells with rounded nuclei which often have a perinuclear 'halo' producing a 'poached-egg' appearance (Fig. 6.6), the tumour cells are often arranged in nodules and show propensity to cluster around neurons

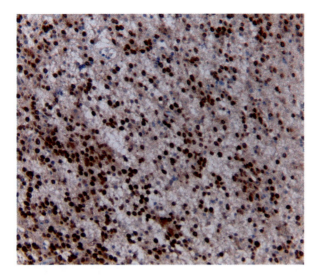

Fig. 6.4 Immunohistochemistry of oligodendroglioma showing a strong cytoplasmic immunore-activity with an antibody to mutant IDH1 protein. Note reactive glial cells are negative

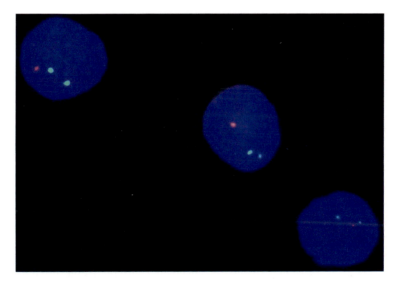

Fig. 6.5 Fluorescent *in situ* hybridisation (FISH) of oligodendroglioma at high magnification, with chromosomal loss indicated by a single copy of chromosome arm 1p (*red*) and two copies of chromosome arm 1q (*green*) in each nucleus

(perineuronal satellitosis). Oligodendrogliomas are WHO Grade II tumours, how-ever, some tumours show increased mitotic activity and cellularity, and are some-times associated with necrosis and vascular proliferation and are termed anaplastic oligodendroglioma (WHO Grade III). If there is an intermingled astrocytic compo-nent, the tumours have traditionally been labelled as either oligoastrocytomas or

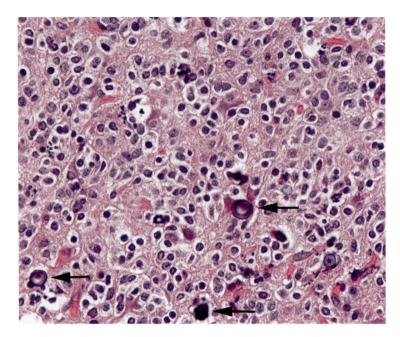

Fig. 6.6 Oligodendroglioma composed of cells with rounded nuclei and areas of perinuclear clearing producing a poached-egg appearance and focal calcification (*arrows*). H&E stain

anaplastic oligoastrocytomas, depending on biological grade. However, genetic sub-typing suggests that almost all mixed tumours can be separated into either astrocytic or oligodendroglial subtypes [6]. Like diffuse astrocytomas, oligodendroglial tumours commonly show mutations in *isocitrate dehydrogenase* (*IDH*) *genes*. Around 70–80 % of oligodendroglial tumours show a characteristic chromosomal translocation, resulting in loss of most of chromosome arms 1p and 19q. Tumours which show this co-deletion have a better prognosis and, in particular, a good response to chemotherapy and radiotherapy.

6.3.3.2 Ependymomas

These glial tumours show evidence of ependymal differentiation, often develop close to the ventricular system, and are common in the posterior fossa in children. Microscopically they show perivascular pseudorosettes (Fig. 6.7) and ependymal tubular structures. Classic ependymomas are WHO Grade II tumours, although tumours showing increased mitotic activity and cellularity, necrosis and vascular proliferation, are termed as anaplastic ependymomas which are WHO Grade III. **Myxopapillary ependymomas** are usually found in the cauda equina region and are well defined sausage-shaped tumours which are WHO Grade I, and if removed intact, have an excellent prognosis. **Subependymomas** occur in adults, within the

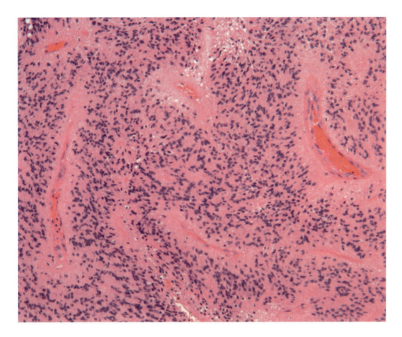

Fig. 6.7 Ependymoma composed of glial cells showing characteristic perivascular pseudorosettes with areas around blood vessels devoid of nuclei. H&E stain

fourth or lateral ventricles and are WHO Grade I tumours which may be asymptomatic and are sometimes discovered incidentally at autopsy.

6.4 Neuronal Tumours With or Without Glial Features

A number of tumours may show evidence of neuronal differentiation, sometimes with areas of glial differentiation. Most of these tumours are relatively low grade and occur in children and young adults, often causing intractable epilepsy.

6.4.1 Gangliocytoma and Ganglioglioma

These are slow growing tumours containing mature ganglionic cells (gangliocytoma, WHO Grade I) (Fig. 6.8), or with an additional astrocytic glial component (ganglioglioma, WHO Grade II). These tumours usually are relatively well circumscribed, and in rare cases of the mixed tumours, the glial component may undergo malignant transformation. They often present with a cyst associated with a mural nodule, particularly in the temporal lobe, and with seizures.

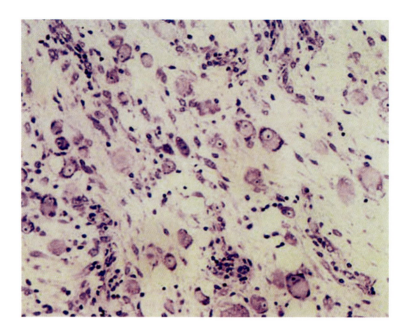

Fig. 6.8 Gangliocytoma composed of haphazardly arranged mature neuronal cells, some of which are multinucleate. Nissl stain

6.4.2 Dysembryoplastic Neuroepithelial Tumour

This tumour, usually labelled as a DNET, is benign (WHO Grade I) and usually presents with drug resistant complex partial seizures under the age of 20 years. They are common in the temporal lobe and have a complex histological pattern with a mixture of neuronal and glial elements, sometimes associated with underlying cortical dysplasia. They have a nodular appearance and do not produce any mass effect on imaging. Surgery may be very effective at treating epilepsy.

6.4.3 Central Neurocytoma

These tumours are WHO Grade II and usually present in young adults with features of raised intracranial pressure and a large enhancing mass within the anterior ventricular system. Histologically they are composed of small uniform neuronal cells which resemble oligodendroglioma cells (Fig. 6.9), but which express neuronal proteins. Despite their size, most central neurocytomas have a relatively good prognosis, however, a small proportion may have anaplastic change and a propensity to recur.

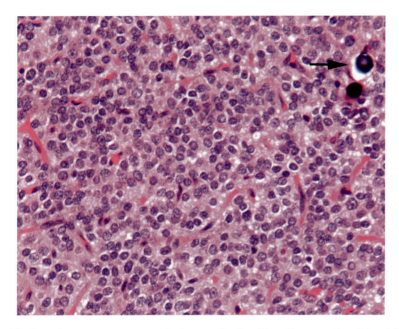

Fig. 6.9 Central neurocytoma composed of neuronal cells with uniform round nuclei and focal calcification (*arrow*), bearing a resemblance to oligodendroglioma. H&E stain

6.4.4 Desmoplastic Infantile Astrocytoma/Ganglioglioma

These are large, often superficial and cystic hemispheric tumours that occur in infants. Some are composed predominantly of a desmoplastic (collagen forming) astrocytic component, but they may also contain ganglionic cells. They are WHO Grade I tumours and have a good prognosis following surgery.

6.4.5 Dysplastic Gangliocytoma of the Cerebellum (Lhermitte-Duclos Syndrome)

This is a hamartomatous lesion of the cerebellum associated with enlarged abnormal neurons and disturbance of the normal cerebellar architecture. However, some lesions can produce mass effect and behave like a benign tumour causing raised intracranial pressure. They may be associated with Cowden's syndrome and other developmental abnormalities of the CNS.

There are a number of other rare neuronal tumours, including a **spinal paraganglioma**, **extraventricular neurocytomas**, **cerebellar liponeurocytomas**, **papillary glioneuronal tumours** and **rosette-forming glioneuronal tumours of the fourth ventricle**.

6.5   Embryonal Tumours

These are neuroepithelial tumours that predominantly occur in childhood and are composed of primitive cells which may show neuronal and other forms of differentiation. Unlike the low-grade neuronal tumours described above, these tumours have a tendency to grow rapidly and may disseminate throughout the CNS via the CSF.

6.5.1   Medulloblastoma

These are WHO Grade IV embryonal tumours arising in the cerebellum, most often in childhood, but also in adults. Most occur sporadically, but they can also occur in the context of Gorlin, Turcot and Li-Fraumeni syndromes. Medulloblastomas show evidence of neuronal differentiation, in the form of Homer Wright rosettes (Fig. 6.10) and production of neuronal proteins, and there are a number of histological subtypes including the classic medulloblastoma, desmoplastic/nodular medulloblastoma, medulloblastoma with extensive nodularity, anaplastic medulloblastoma and large cell medulloblastoma. The latter two have a more aggressive behaviour.

A number of genetic changes have been described in medulloblastomas, including isochromosome 17q, alterations in both the sonic hedgehog (SHH) and the wingless (WNT) pathways. Around 10 % of medulloblastomas have WNT alterations, mostly those of the classic histology, and this subgroup has an excellent prognosis.

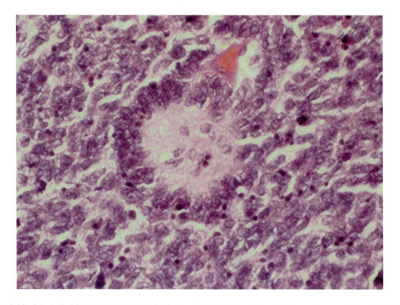

Fig. 6.10 Medulloblastoma composed of closely packed cells with irregular nuclei, mitotic figures and forming a large Homer Wright rosette. H&E stain

6.5.2   Primitive Neuroectodermal Tumour

These are tumours which have a similar histological appearance to medulloblastomas, but occur within the cerebral hemispheres (and are a separate entity to the primitive neuroectodermal tumours that arise outside of the CNS). These are WHO Grade IV tumours and may be calcified on imaging. They predominantly occur in children and tend to have a worse prognosis than medulloblastomas. Variants include **neuroblastoma, ganglioneuroblastoma, medulloepitheliomas, ependymoblastoma** and the recently described **embryonal tumour with abundant neuropil and true rosettes (ETANTR)**.

6.5.3   Atypical Teratoid/Rhabdoid Tumour

This is an aggressive (WHO Grade IV) tumour, predominantly of early childhood, that may occur in the cerebral hemispheres and posterior fossa. The tumour is characterised by inactivation of the *INI1 gene*, and is composed of cells which resemble primitive muscle cells (rhabdoid cells) and may show glial or neuronal, epithelial and mesenchymal differentiation.

6.6   Pineal Region Tumours

These occur in both children and adults and often present with raised intracranial pressure, due to aqueduct compression, or brain stem signs, such as Parinaud's syndrome.

Pineal parenchymal tumours range from the relatively slow growing **pineocytomas** (WHO Grade II), to the more aggressive **pineoblastomas** (WHO Grade IV). The latter tumours tend to occur in childhood and have a similar morphological appearance and behaviour to the embryonal tumours described above. An intermediate form of pineal parenchymal tumour also may occur. Benign cysts and a rare **papillary tumour of the pineal region** may also occur.

Although **germ cell tumours** occur at several sites within the CNS, the most common site is the pineal region, particularly during the teenage years. Germ cell tumours have a range in histological subtype including germinomas, embryonal carcinomas, yolk sac tumours, choriocarcinomas and teratomas. Germ cell tumours show variable responses to chemotherapy and radiotherapy.

6.7   Choroid Plexus Tumours

These include the benign **choroid plexus papilloma** and the highly aggressive **choroid plexus carcinoma**. They commonly occur in the fourth or lateral ventricles and cause hydrocephalus, usually due to obstruction of CSF pathways, but rarely due to overproduction of CSF. Choroid plexus carcinomas are largely confined to young children, whereas papillomas occur in both children and adults.

6.8   Meningeal Tumours

6.8.1   Meningiomas

Meningiomas are relatively common tumours arising from arachnoidal cells, and although many are symptomatic, some are discovered incidentally and may grow extremely slowly. In about 10 % of cases, meningiomas are multiple, and this is more common in familial tumour syndromes such as neurofibromatosis type 2. Meningiomas are uncommon in childhood and there is an overall female predominance, which is particularly marked for spinal tumours. Common sites include the convexities, the falx, olfactory groove, sphenoid ridge, petrous ridge and tentorium, but they may occur at other sites including within the ventricular system. Meningiomas are attached to (Fig. 6.11a), and commonly invade, dura and may invade the overlying bone (causing hyperostosis), in some cases protruding through into subcutaneous tissues of the scalp. On imaging they are often isodense with brain, show calcification and usually show uniform contrast enhancement. Histologically there are many different subtypes, but most are characterised by the presence of whorl formation (Fig. 6.11b), and the majority are WHO Grade I tumours. Around 20 % tumours are WHO Grade II, with an increased propensity to recur, and these include tumours with increased mitotic activity (atypical meningiomas), brain invasion (Fig. 6.11c), chordoid or clear cell morphology. About 3 % tumours have a very high mitotic rate, anaplastic cytology (which may resemble a carcinoma or sarcoma), papillary or rhabdoid morphology, and are classed as WHO Grade III tumours, almost all of which will recur. Occasionally WHO Grade III meningiomas metastasise outside of the CNS, particularly following surgery. Embolisation prior to surgery can cause tumour necrosis and increased mitotic activity complicating histological interpretation.

The aetiology of most meningiomas is unknown although radiation is a recognised risk factor. About half of meningiomas show loss of merlin, often due to monosomy of chromosome 22 and mutations in the other copy of the *neurofibromatosis type 2 gene*, *merlin* (Box 6.1), and many of the remaining meningiomas have mutations in other genes including *TRAF7, AKT1, SMO, SMARCE1* and *KLF4* [7, 8]. Meningiomas without merlin loss are more likely to occur in the subfrontal region, to be of meningothelial and secretory subtypes, and less likely to be histologically aggressive [7–9].

Box 6.1 Merlin

Product of NF2 gene (also known as schwannomin) on chromosome arm 22q. Germ-line loss occurs in NF2.

Roles at cell membrane and nucleus in control of cytoskeleton, cell-cell interactions and growth.

Loss seen in schwannomas and many meningiomas and ependymomas.

6.8.2 Other Tumours of the Meninges

In addition to meningiomas, a wide range of benign and malignant soft tissue tumours may arise from the meninges. These include benign tumours of fat (**lipoma**) which may include a prominent vascular component (**angiolipoma**), the latter

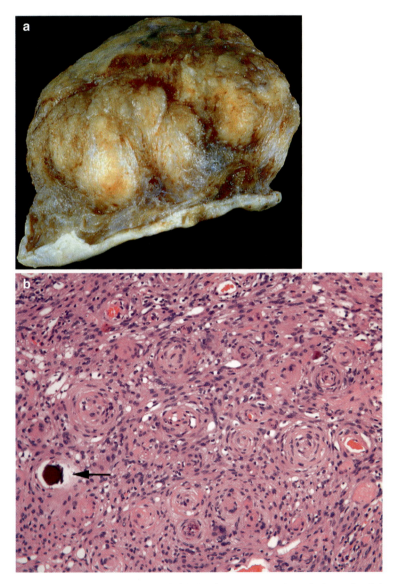

Fig. 6.11 (**a**) Meningioma having a smooth lobulated appearance and attached to strip of dura. (**b**) Microscopically forming characteristic whorls with a calcified psammoma body (*arrow*). (**c**) Meningioma showing upwards 'finger-like' brain invasion, increasing the likelihood of local recurrence. H&E stain

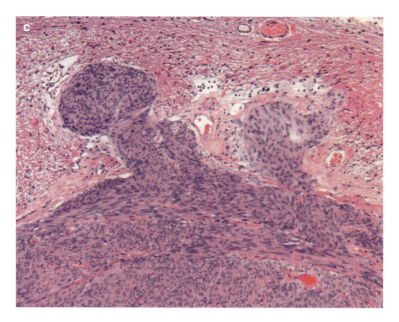

Fig. 6.11 (continued)

showing a propensity for the thoracic spinal region. **Solitary fibrous tumours** and **haemangiopericytomas** have a similar appearance on imaging to meningiomas, however, these may also arise outside of the CNS, and presumably do not derive from arachnoidal cells. Haemangiopericytomas have a higher rate of recurrence than most meningiomas. Both benign and malignant **melanocytic tumours** may arise from the meninges. **Haemangioblastomas** are benign tumours, which most commonly occur in the cerebellum and on imaging typically have a cyst with a contrast-enhancing nodule in the wall. They usually have a leptomeningeal attachment and histologically are composed of lipid-filled stromal cells surrounded by a rich vascular network (Fig. 6.12). Many are sporadic, however, significant minority occur in the context of von Hippel-Lindau syndrome. Most sporadic tumours occur in the cerebellum, however, in the context of von Hippel-Lindau syndrome may occur earlier, in the cerebral hemispheres and spinal cord, and may be multiple.

6.9 Pituitary Region Tumours

Pituitary adenomas are relatively common benign tumours of the anterior pituitary gland (adenohypophysis). These may present with mass effect, causing visual disturbance from compression of the overlying optic chiasm, but may also present with endocrine symptoms due to over production of a pituitary hormone. Many are clinically non-functioning, although many of these latter tumours show immunohistochemical evidence of gonadotropin production. Prolactinomas may cause amenorrhoea and

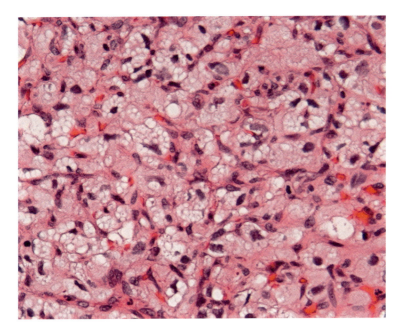

Fig. 6.12 Haemangioblastoma composed of stromal cells with irregular dark nuclei and abundant vacuolated lipid-filled cytoplasm separated by numerous small capillaries. H&E stain

reduced fertility in women, growth hormone producing tumours may cause acromegaly and gigantism, ACTH-producing tumours result in Cushing's syndrome and TSH-producing tumours may cause hyperthyroidism. Subclassification of pituitary adenomas has become more complex [10], and involves the use of immunohisto-chemistry to detect the presence of hormones (which may not be endocrinologically active) and transcription factors, and may allow subtyping into tumours which have a high density of hormone (densely granulated) and low density (sparsely granulated). It has become evident that certain histological subtypes including TSH-producing adenomas, the sparsely granulated ACTH-producing macroadenoma, and relatively uncommon acidophil stem cell adenoma, silent subtype III adenoma and Crooke cell adenoma, may behave more aggressively with a higher rate of local invasion and recurrence. Pituitary apoplexy may be caused by haemorrhage into a tumour resulting in visual loss, and requires urgent surgical decompression.

Pituitary carcinomas are very uncommon tumours that by definition have spread within and/or outside of the CNS, and are usually endocrinologically active. Histologically pituitary carcinomas range from a relatively benign appearance, to frankly malignant, and have to be distinguished from systemic carcinomas, which have metastasised to the pituitary.

Rarer benign tumours of the pituitary gland arising from the neurohypophysis include the **granular cell tumour** and **pituicytoma** and, from the adenohypohysis, the **spindle cell oncocytoma**.

Not all masses within the pituitary gland are tumours; **Rathke's cleft cysts** derived from embryological remnants are relatively common, and **lymphocytic**

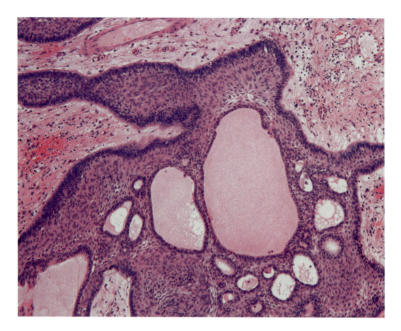

Fig. 6.13 Craniopharyngioma composed of sheets of cohesive epithelial cells forming cystic spaces. H&E stain

hypophysitis is an inflammatory condition, particularly common in late pregnancy, that may cause pituitary enlargement and pituitary insufficiency.

Craniopharyngiomas usually occur in the suprasellar region and occur in both children and adults. They are composed of epithelial cells and often form areas of cystic change and calcify (Fig. 6.13). There are two histological variants (adamantinomatous and papillary) and although are relatively slow growing have a high tendency to recur following surgery.

A number of other lesions may occur in the pituitary region including meningiomas, germ cell tumours, Langerhan's cell histiocytosis, chordomas, astrocytic tumours and metastatic carcinoma.

6.10   Lymphomas

Lymphomas occur within the CNS either as primary lymphomas or extra-CNS tumours, which have spread. The vast majority of primary CNS lymphomas are high grade diffuse B-cell lymphomas which often occur in a periventricular distribution. They may show dramatic transient response to steroid treatment, which can result in a non-diagnostic biopsy, although probably not in the majority of cases [11]. Some of these tumours are associated with Epstein-Barr virus reactivation, particularly lymphomas occurring in immunocompromised individuals. T-cell lymphomas are rare in the CNS. Plasma cell tumours and multiple myeloma are

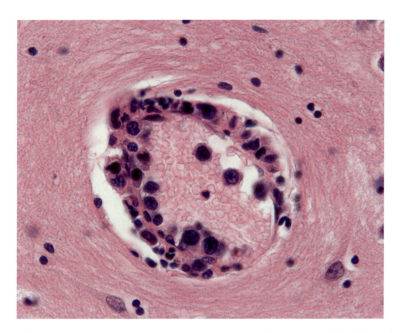

Fig. 6.14 Intravascular lymphoma showing irregular neoplastic lymphoid cells within a blood vessel of brain. H&E stain

common in the paraspinal region. Many systemic lymphomas may spread to the CNS, but Hodgkin's lymphoma only very rarely does.

A condition that is particularly difficult to diagnose during life is intravascular B-cell lymphoma (also known as angiotropic lymphoma) (Fig. 6.14). This affects multiple organs/tissues in the body, but often produces CNS symptoms related to vascular occlusion. A useful clue to the diagnosis is raised serum lactate dehydrogenase, but diagnosis depends on a tissue and can sometimes be made with a skin, bone marrow or muscle biopsy. However, often this diagnosis is made at autopsy.

6.11   Tumours of the Peripheral Nerves

These tumours commonly known as nerve sheath tumours are comprised predominantly of schwannomas and neurofibromas. Both are benign (WHO Grade I) tumours composed of neoplastic schwann cells.

Schwannomas consist of a clonal population of schwann cells, usually arising eccentrically attached to a peripheral nerve and show classic biphasic histological features with compact cellular areas (Antoni-A tissue), where there is often nuclear alignment, (Verocay body formation) (Fig. 6.15a), along with other areas of loosely textured tissue with lipidised cells (Antoni-B tissue), which often contain degenerate blood vessels and show cystic change. These tumours may occur on any peripheral nerve, but within the cranial cavity most commonly arise from the vestibular portion of the eighth cranial nerve (acoustic neuroma) resulting in hearing loss (Fig. 6.15b). Schwannomas may be multiple, particularly in the context of neurofibromatosis type 2 and schwannomatosis. **Plexiform schwannomas** often have the appearance of bundles of rope and some tumours are pigmented (**melanotic schwannomas**) and these latter lesions tend to have a more aggressive behaviour and may occur in the context of Carney's complex. Generally however, schwannomas only very rarely undergo malignant transformation.

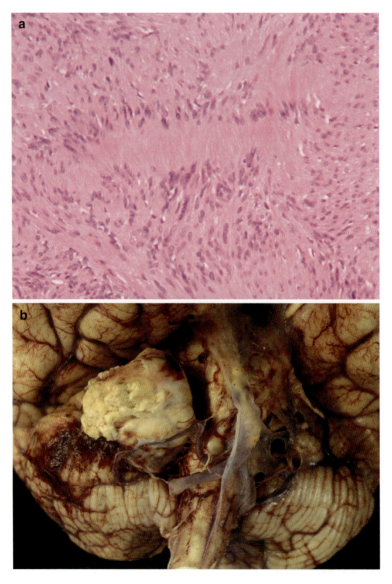

Fig. 6.15 (a) Schwannoma composed of spindle shaped cells showing central areas of nuclear alignment, forming a Verocay body. H&E stain. (b) Schwannoma of vestibular nerve forming a yellow mass at the cerebellopontine angle and indenting the pons

Neurofibromas result in diffuse expansion of a nerve and, in addition to the neoplastic schwann cells, often contain other cell types including fibroblasts. These usually occur on one or more peripheral nerves and may form plexiform lesions, particularly in the context of neurofibromatosis type 1. Neurofibromas can undergo malignant transformation to form **malignant peripheral nerve sheath tumours** (WHO Grade II, III or IV), although these tumours may also arise *de novo*. **Perineuriomas** are rare, usually benign, tumours of the peripheral nerve.

6.12   Other Tumours Affecting the CNS

Any systemic malignant tumour may spread to the CNS, particularly carcinomas. **Adenocarcinomas** more commonly spread than squamous carcinomas and some primary tumours in particular, such as breast, lung and renal cell carcinomas, spread relatively commonly. **Malignant melanoma** should also be considered, particularly in younger individuals and those presenting with haemorrhage. Individuals with systemic tumours may also develop an autoimmune paraneoplastic disorder causing an encephalomyelitis or cerebellar degeneration.

A range of cysts may also occur within the CNS, which are usually benign and of developmental origin. These include **epidermoid cysts** commonly occurring in the cerebello-pontine angle, **colloid cysts of the third ventricle** (Fig. 6.16) and **arachnoidal cysts** derived from the leptomeninges.

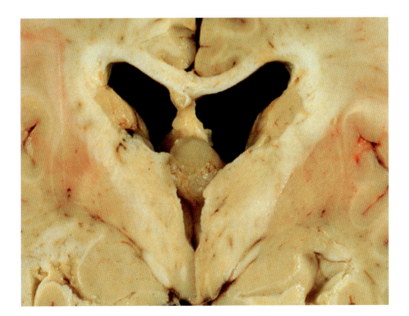

Fig. 6.16 Colloid cyst of the third ventricle forming a grape-like structure, which may intermittently occlude CSF flow and cause acute hydrocephalus

References

1. Pobereskin LH, Chadduck JB. Incidence of brain tumours in two English counties: a population based study. J Neurol Neurosurg Psychiatry. 2000;69(4):464–71.
2. Louis DN, Ohgaki H, Wiestler OD, Cavenee W. WHO classification of tumours of the central nervous system. 4th ed. Lyon: International Agency for Research on Cancer; 2007.
3. Hardell L, Carlberg M, Soderqvist F, Mild KH. Case–control study of the association between malignant brain tumours diagnosed between 2007 and 2009 and mobile and cordless phone use. Int J Oncol. 2013;43(6):1833–45.
4. Benson VS, Pirie K, Schuz J, Reeves GK, Beral V, Green J, et al. Mobile phone use and risk of brain neoplasms and other cancers: prospective study. Int J Epidemiol. 2013;42(3): 792–802.
5. Barresi V, Branca G, Granata F, Alafaci C, Caffo M, Tuccari G. Embolized meningiomas: risk of overgrading and neo-angiogenesis. J Neurooncol. 2013;113(2):207–19.
6. Sahm F, Reuss D, Koelsche C, Capper D, Schittenhelm J, Heim S, et al. Farewell to oligoastrocytoma: in situ molecular genetics favor classification as either oligodendroglioma or astrocytoma. Acta Neuropathol. 2014;128(4):551–9.
7. Clark VE, Erson-Omay EZ, Serin A, Yin J, Cotney J, Ozduman K, et al. Genomic analysis of non-NF2 meningiomas reveals mutations in TRAF7, KLF4, AKT1, and SMO. Science. 2013;339(6123):1077–80.
8. Brastianos PK, Horowitz PM, Santagata S, Jones RT, McKenna A, Getz G, et al. Genomic sequencing of meningiomas identifies oncogenic SMO and AKT1 mutations. Nat Genet. 2013;45(3):285–9.
9. Kros J, de Greve K, van Tilborg A, Hop W, Pieterman H, Avezaat C, et al. NF2 status of meningiomas is associated with tumour localization and histology. J Pathol. 2001;194(3):367–72.
10. Mete O, Asa SL. Clinicopathological correlations in pituitary adenomas. Brain Pathol. 2012;22(4):443–53.
11. Porter AB, Giannini C, Kaufmann T, Lucchinetti CF, Wu W, Decker PA, et al. Primary central nervous system lymphoma can be histologically diagnosed after previous corticosteroid use: a pilot study to determine whether corticosteroids prevent the diagnosis of primary central nervous system lymphoma. Ann Neurol. 2008;63(5):662–7.

Chapter 7
Demyelinating Diseases

Abstract Demyelinating diseases are characterised by the loss of myelin with relative axonal preservation, and affect both the central and peripheral nervous systems.
The most common primary demyelinating disease of the central nervous system is
multiple sclerosis, which can be classified into different clinical and pathological subtypes. The pathology of the other demyelinating diseases affecting the central nervous
system, including Devic's disease, acute disseminated encephalomyelitis and acute
haemorrhagic leukoencephalopathy, is also described. The pathology of trigeminal
neuralgia is briefly discussed as it involves demyelination of the nerve root.

Keywords Demyelination • Plaques • Multiple sclerosis • Remyelination

Demyelinating disorders are characterised pathologically by loss of myelin with *relative*
preservation of axons. They may affect either the peripheral or central nervous system
(CNS), and in a few conditions e.g. adrenoleukodystrophies, affect both. Disorders
affecting the peripheral nerves are discussed in Chap. 10. In addition to 'primary' demyelinating disorders, demyelination may be caused by infectious, metabolic and toxic factors and each of these will be discussed in their relevant chapters. This chapter will focus
on primary demyelinating disorders affecting the CNS, but not include disorders of failure to produce myelin such as the leukodystrophies, which are covered in Chap. 14.

7.1 Multiple Sclerosis

Multiple sclerosis (MS) is by far the commonest demyelinating disorder of the CNS,
affecting both the brain and spinal cord, usually presenting in young adulthood and is
more frequent in women than men. There are a wide variety of clinical features including upper motor neuron weakness, paraesthesia, proprioceptive loss, cerebellar signs,
vertigo, diplopia and vomiting. The disease is often preceded by an episode of optic
neuritis and may also result in bladder and bowel disturbance, trigeminal neuralgia
and cognitive impairment. Useful abnormal investigations which support the diagnosis include oligoclonal bands of IgG within the CSF, delayed visual evoked responses
and enhancing areas of the white matter on magnetic resonance imaging of the CNS.

© Springer International Publishing Switzerland 2015
D.A. Hilton, A.G. Shivane, *Neuropathology Simplified: A Guide for Clinicians
and Neuroscientists*, DOI 10.1007/978-3-319-14605-8_7

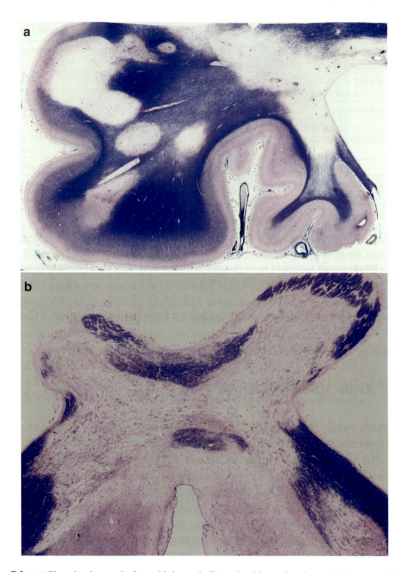

Fig. 7.2 (**a**) Chronic plaques in frontal lobe and, (**b**) optic chiasm showing well demarcated areas lacking myelin. Myelin stain

7.2 Neuromyelitis Optica (Devic's Disease)

Neuromyelitis optica is the association of optic neuritis, usually with visual loss, and transverse myelitis, within a few weeks of each other. This condition has sufficient differences from classic MS to be regarded as a separate entity. In most patients the visual loss occurs first, followed by paraplegia, sensory loss, bladder and bowel disturbance. There are usually few or no lesions in the brain elsewhere, and the

Table 7.2 Types of MS plaque

Active plaque	Active demyelination with an infiltrate of lymphocytes and macrophages, many of which contain lipid, and reactive astrocytes (Fig. 7.3). Extensive loss of myelin with good preservation of axons.
Chronic active plaque	Area of demyelination with chronic inflammatory cells around the margin, but no active demyelination
Chronic inactive plaque	Hypocellular gliotic area of demyelination, with loss of oligodendrocytes, and often depletion of axons. No inflammation
Shadow plaque	An area with partial loss of myelin staining (Fig. 7.4). This may include a central area of demyelination with a border of intermediate myelin preservation, or the entire lesion may show partial myelin staining. These lesions result from remyelination, usually mediated by oligodendrocytes, but in the brain stem and spinal cord they may be mediated by Schwann cells.
Grey matter plaque	Area of well defined myelin loss within the grey matter, which in the cortex may be subpial, intracortical or involve the cortex and adjacent white matter (Fig. 7.5). Often inflammation in adjacent leptomeninges. There may be activated microglia within these lesions, but macrophages and lymphocytes are usually absent. Best identified histologically using immunohistochemistry with an antibody to myelin basic protein.

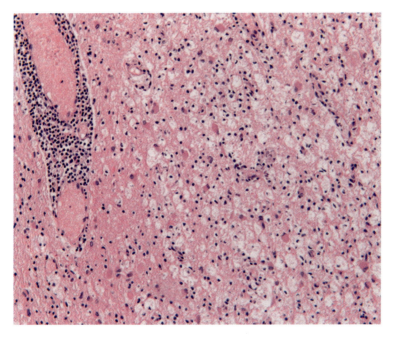

Fig. 7.3 Histological appearances of active plaque with numerous inflammatory cells including perivascular lymphocytes, reactive astrocytes and macrophages containing myelin debris. H&E stain

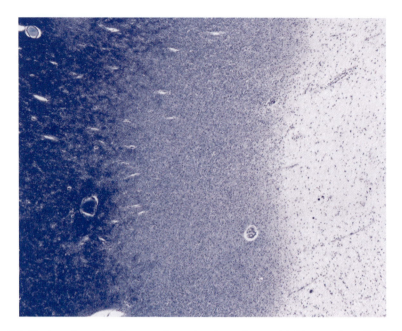

Fig. 7.4 Shadow plaque showing area of complete demyelination (*right*), normal myelin (*left*) and intermediate zone or 'shadow' indicating partial remyelination. Myelin stain

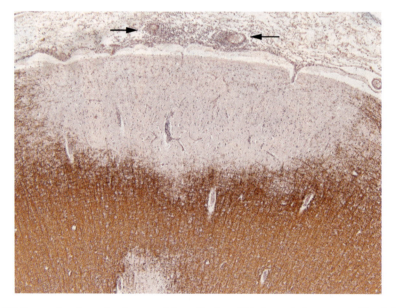

Fig. 7.5 Grey matter plaque showing area of demyelination within the cortical grey matter. Note inflammation in overlying leptomeninges (*between arrows*). Immunohistochemistry for myelin basic protein

spinal cord involvement usually includes a contiguous segment extending for 3 or more vertebral segments (which is unusual in MS). The majority of patients have an antibody in the serum directed against aquaporin 4 [4], which is a water channel expressed highly in astrocytic end-feet. The optic nerves and spinal cord show extensive demyelination, but in addition may be oedematous and necrotic. The inflammatory infiltrates include relatively few lymphocytes and more perivascular neutrophils and eosinophils, with prominent perivascular deposition of immuno-globulins and activated complement associated with fibrosis of blood vessels. The lesions in the spinal cord are often centrally located. Oligoclonal bands are not normally present in the CSF.

7.3 Acute Disseminated Encephalomyelitis (ADEM)

This is an acute inflammatory demyelinating disorder of the CNS which often follows an infectious disease or vaccination by several days to weeks. Presentation is usually with headache, vomiting, fever and neurological impairment. The disorder may follow a wide range of infectious disorders and is more common in young children and adolescents. It is often monophasic and responds to immunosuppressive treatment, however, some cases are fatal or are left with persistent neurological deficits, and a few may develop relapses (multiphasic disseminated encephalomyelitis) [5]. Oligoclonal bands may be present in some cases and imaging may show multiple areas of signal abnormality, particularly in the subcortical white matter with relative sparing of the periventricular regions. The lesions may be rather ill-defined to the naked eye and there may be brain swelling. The characteristic lesions are serpiginous areas of perivenous demyelination (Fig. 7.6), with foamy macrophages containing myelin debris, and relatively few lymphocytes and reactive astrocytes.

7.4 Acute Haemorrhagic Leukoencephalopathy

This is usually a fatal disorder characterised by fever, neck stiffness and neurological deficit leading to death within a few days. Seizures may be prominent, and both adults and children are affected. Cases are usually preceded by a febrile illness, such as an upper respiratory tract infection, but may also follow episodes of inflammatory bowel disease, septicaemia and some toxins. The brain is congested and swollen and contains multiple petechial haemorrhages throughout the white matter (Fig. 7.7) including the brainstem, cerebellum and spinal cord. Histologically, there are areas of perivascular demyelination associated with haemorrhage and fibrinoid necrosis of vessel walls.

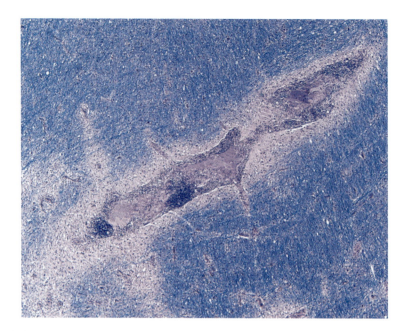

Fig. 7.6 Acute disseminated encephalomyelitis showing serpiginous area of demyelination adjacent to blood vessel. Myelin stain

Fig. 7.7 Acute haemorrhagic
leukoencephalopathy
showing multiple petechial
haemorrhages in white matter

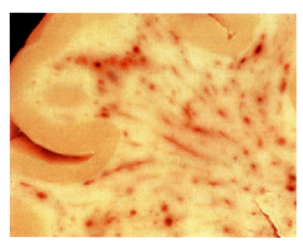

7.5 Trigeminal Neuralgia

The majority of cases of trigeminal neuralgia are associated with vascular compression of the trigeminal nerve root. This has been shown to result in demyelination in the central portion of the nerve root and closely apposed 'naked' axons, sometimes with aberrant remyelination [6]. These pathological features are believed to underlie the episodes of sensory disturbance, due to ephaptic transmission or 'cross talk', between nerve fibres. Trigeminal neuralgia is also seen in cases of multiple sclerosis and nerve root compression secondary to a space-occupying lesion. Other syndromes affecting cranial nerves are also associated with vascular nerve root compression and may have a similar pathology.

References

1. Lublin FD, Reingold SC, Cohen JA, Cutter GR, Sorensen PS, Thompson AJ, et al. Defining the clinical course of multiple sclerosis: the 2013 revisions. Neurology. 2014;83(3):278–86.
2. Popescu BF, Lucchinetti CF. Meningeal and cortical grey matter pathology in multiple sclerosis. BMC Neurol. 2012;12:11.
3. Lucchinetti CF, Gavrilova RH, Metz I, Parisi JE, Scheithauer BW, Weigand S, et al. Clinical and radiographic spectrum of pathologically confirmed tumefactive multiple sclerosis. Brain. 2008;131(Pt 7):1759–75.
4. Lennon VA, Wingerchuk DM, Kryzer TJ, Pittock SJ, Lucchinetti CF, Fujihara K, et al. A serum autoantibody marker of neuromyelitis optica: distinction from multiple sclerosis. Lancet. 2004;364(9451):2106–12.
5. Dale RC, de Sousa C, Chong WK, Cox TC, Harding B, Neville BG. Acute disseminated encephalomyelitis, multiphasic disseminated encephalomyelitis and multiple sclerosis in children. Brain. 2000;123(Pt 12):2407–22.
6. Love S, Hilton DA, Coakham HB. Central demyelination of the Vth nerve root in trigeminal neuralgia associated with vascular compression. Brain Pathol. 1998;8(1):1–11; discussion 11–2.

Chapter 8
Epilepsy

Abstract Epilepsy is a common neurological disorder affecting all age groups. Any lesion within the brain can be potentially epileptogenic and therefore, causes for epilepsy are varied and include malformations, tumours, vascular disease, inflammatory and infectious diseases, metabolic diseases, trauma and rarely neuro-degenerative conditions. This chapter deals with some of the more common causes of epilepsy and their neuropathology. There is a greater risk of sudden death in patients with epilepsy compared to the general population. The neuropathology of sudden unexpected death in epilepsy (SUDEP) is briefly discussed.

Keywords Epilepsy • Seizure • Cortical dysplasia • Hippocampal sclerosis • SUDEP

Epilepsy a common neurological disorder which affects 1–2 % of the population world-wide, forming a heterogeneous group of diseases in which there is a tendency for recurrent seizures. A seizure results from an uncontrolled sustained discharge of a large group of neurons within the brain and can be of two major types: generalised (tonic-clonic, atonic, myoclonic, absence) or focal/partial seizures (simple or complex partial). In children, generalised seizures are more common, whereas partial seizures are the predominant seizure type in adults. Most seizures are self-limiting, but in some instances they can persist for longer than 30 min (*status epilepticus*, which is a medical emergency).

There are various causes and predisposing factors for epilepsy (Table 8.1). In majority of cases of epilepsy there is no identifiable cause (*idiopathic epilepsy*). Around 30 % of patients have a close relative with epilepsy suggesting a strong genetic component. Several types of epilepsy, earlier considered to be idiopathic, have now shown gene mutations involving the voltage-or ligand-gated ion channels (e.g. sodium, potassium and calcium channels, nicotinic and GABA receptors).

The investigation in a case of new-onset epilepsy involves identifying the cause for epilepsy and includes: routine blood analysis (for haematopoietic, hepatic and renal function), electrocardiogram, electroencephalogram and neuroimaging. These guide further management in individual patients. In most cases, the seizures are well

© Springer International Publishing Switzerland 2015   113
D.A. Hilton, A.G. Shivane, *Neuropathology Simplified: A Guide for Clinicians and Neuroscientists*, DOI 10.1007/978-3-319-14605-8_8

Table 8.1 Epilepsy: causes and predisposing factors

Cortical abnormalities (*Focal cortical dysplasia, Hippocampal sclerosis*)
Brain tumours (*both primary and secondary; e.g. DNET and other low-grade glioneuronal tumours*)
Trauma ('*Post-traumatic epilepsy*')
Cerebrovascular disease (*Vascular malformations, Stroke*)
Inflammatory diseases (*Rasmussen's encephalitis*)
Infections (e.g. *Herpes encephalitis, Malaria, Cysticercosis*)
Neurodegenerative diseases (*Lafora body disease, Creutzfeldt-Jakob disease, Alzheimer's disease*)
Metabolic diseases (*Lysosomal storage diseases, Electrolyte imbalance, Uraemia, Alcohol abuse*)

controlled with anti-epileptic drugs, but surgery is considered in cases having structural lesions such as low grade neoplasms or cortical dysplasia which are generally refractory to drugs.

8.1 Rasmussen's Encephalitis

Rasmussen's encephalitis is a rare progressive seizure disorder of unknown aetiology, commonly presenting in childhood. It begins with partial motor seizures, secondary generalised seizures or epilepsia partialis continua and is associated with neurological deficits and unilateral hemispheric atrophy. The macroscopic brain changes are subtle and predominantly unilateral and include cerebral atrophy and mildly discoloured cortex. The histology in early stages shows an inflammatory process consisting of mainly T lymphocytes around blood vessels, microglial reaction and neuronophagia. These features are similar to those seen in viral encephalitis which needs to be excluded by appropriate tests. At a later stage, there is pan-cortical neuronal loss, gliosis and spongiosis with minimal inflammation. The inflammatory process is multifocal, patchy, and although unilateral in most cases, occasional post-mortem cases with bilateral pathology have been described. There is no convincing evidence of an infectious aetiology [1] and some evidence suggests that this represents an immunological disease [2]. There can be associated lesions such as focal cortical dysplasia, vascular malformation, and tumours. Early treatment with immunosuppression or surgery (hemispherectomy) may be effective in slowing the disease progression and controlling seizures.

8.2 Focal Cortical Dysplasia

Focal cortical dysplasia (FCD) represents a malformative lesion arising from an abnormal cortical development (the term 'dysplasia' in this context should not be mistaken for a premalignant condition). FCD is frequently associated with epilepsy

Table 8.2 Classification of focal cortical dysplasia

Type I (isolated)	Type II (isolated)	Type III (associated with principal lesion)
Abnormal cortical lamination	Dysmorphic neurons and balloon cells (IIb)	Hippocampal sclerosis
		Glial or glioneuronal tumour
		Vascular malformation
		Others (trauma, ischaemia, encephalitis)

(usually refractory to drugs), in both children and adults. The lesions are commonly located within the frontal or temporal lobes and may be visible as focally thickened cortex or blurred grey-white matter junction on naked eye inspection. The International League Against Epilepsy (ILAE) task force has introduced a three-tiered consensus classification system based largely on neuropathological features (Table 8.2) [3].

FCD type I is characterised by abnormalities in the lamination of cerebral cortex (a normal cerebral cortex has six well defined layers, see Chap. 1). The abnormal lamination can be either radial/vertical (Ia), tangential/horizontal (Ib) or both (Ic) and can be present in one or several lobes. These lesions can be detected on MRI scans. FCD type II has cytologic abnormalities in addition to abnormal lamination. They contain dysmorphic neurons (IIa) or dysmorphic neurons and balloon cells (large cell body, glassy pink cytoplasm and no Nissl substance) (IIb). FCD IIb can be recognised on MRI scans ('*transmantle sign*' or funnel-like signal change). FCD III refers to cortical lamination abnormalities associated with a principal lesion such as hippocampal sclerosis (IIIa), tumours (IIIb), vascular malformations (IIIc) and other lesions acquired during early life (trauma, ischaemia, inflammatory, infections; IIId).

8.3 Hippocampal Sclerosis

Hippocampal sclerosis (also known as 'Ammon's horn sclerosis' or 'Mesial temporal sclerosis') is commonly seen in temporal lobe resections for intractable epilepsy and also in post-mortem brains of epilepsy-related deaths. The exact cause of hippocampal sclerosis is not known, but is presumed to be acquired and multifactorial. A brain insult during early life (such as febrile convulsion) may be the initiating event in some cases for progressive hippocampal damage. The role of other factors such as genes, inflammation and developmental processes is beginning to be understood [4].

The pathology of hippocampal sclerosis is characterised by specific patterns of neuronal loss and gliosis. This is depicted in the recent consensus classification [5] which categorises hippocampal sclerosis into typical (type 1) and atypical (types 2 and 3). Macroscopically, the affected hippocampus may appear firm and reduced in

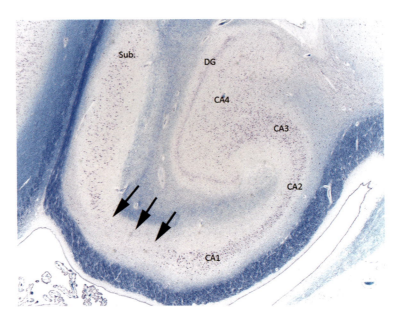

Fig. 8.1 Hippocampal sclerosis from a case of chronic epilepsy showing characteristic neuronal loss in part of CA1 region/Sommer sector (*arrows*). *DG* dentate gyrus, *Sub* subiculum. LFB/CV stain

size with corresponding dilatation of the temporal horn of the lateral ventricle. The histology in a typical case (type 1) shows neuronal loss involving the CA1, CA4/end folium, and CA3 regions (CA2 spared), associated gliosis, dispersion of granule cells within dentate gyrus and scattered hypertrophic neurons in CA4/hilum. In the atypical forms the neuronal loss and gliosis is limited to CA1 (type 2) (Fig. 8.1) or CA4/end folium (type 3). Temporal lobe resections are commonly performed for intractable epilepsy which achieves seizure-free outcome in around 75 % (first 2–3 years after surgery) and 57 % (at 5 years) of patients [6].

8.4   Sudden Unexpected Death in Epilepsy (SUDEP)

Epilepsy patients have two to three times higher standardised mortality rates and are at a greater risk of sudden and premature death compared to the general population [7]. This could be due to the direct effect of seizure itself (status epilepticus, trauma, drowning, aspiration or sudden and unexpected) or due to the underlying disease causing epilepsy. SUDEP is defined as '*Sudden, unexpected, witnessed or unwitnessed, non-traumatic and non-drowning death in patients with epilepsy, with or without evidence for a seizure and excluding documented status epilepticus, in which post-mortem examination does not reveal a toxicologic or anatomic cause for death*' [8]. SUDEP is more common in young adults and in those who are less compliant with anti-convulsant medications. Other risk factors include generalised

Table 8.3 Neuropathological changes in patients with chronic epilepsy

Secondary (acquired) changes due to effect of chronic seizures
Neuronal loss and gliosis (hippocampus, amygdala, cerebral cortex, thalamus, cerebellum)
Leptomeningeal thickening/fibrosis
Excess corpora amylacea in the leptomeninges and white matter
Sub-pial superficial (Chaslin's) gliosis
Vascular hyalinisation and perivascular atrophy of temporal white matter
Other pathologies
Cerebral contusions, oedema, old gliotic scars, hippocampal sclerosis, cerebellar atrophy/ neuronal loss (drugs such as phenytoin)
Cause for epilepsy such as tumours, FCD etc.

tonic-clonic seizures, severe or poorly controlled seizures, nocturnal or unwitnessed seizures, abrupt or frequent change in drugs/dosages and alcohol abuse. Central depression of respiration and/or cardiac arrhythmias occurring during or shortly after a seizure has been postulated, but the exact mechanism of death in SUDEP is still uncertain. The autopsy examination should be full and thorough and include detailed brain examination, histology of major organs (heart and lungs, to exclude a microscopic disease e.g. myocarditis) and toxicology (for anti-convulsant drugs, illicit drugs, and alcohol). The neuropathological examination may reveal evidence of previous seizures (Table 8.3), other pathologies (such as mild cerebral oedema, focal contusions, old gliotic scars, hippocampal sclerosis or cerebellar neuronal loss) or a cause for epilepsy (such as a neoplasm).

References

1. Bien CG, Granata T, Antozzi C, Cross JH, Dulac O, Kurthen M, et al. Pathogenesis, diagnosis and treatment of Rasmussen encephalitis: a European consensus statement. Brain. 2005;128(Pt 3):454–71.
2. Rogers SW, Andrews PI, Gahring LC, Whisenand T, Cauley K, Crain B, et al. Autoantibodies to glutamate receptor GluR3 in Rasmussen's encephalitis. Science. 1994;265(5172):648–51.
3. Blumcke I, Thom M, Aronica E, Armstrong DD, Vinters HV, Palmini A, et al. The clinico-pathologic spectrum of focal cortical dysplasias: a consensus classification proposed by an ad hoc Task Force of the ILAE Diagnostic Methods Commission. Epilepsia. 2011;52(1):158–74.
4. Thom M. Review: hippocampal sclerosis in epilepsy: a neuropathology review. Neuropathol Appl Neurobiol. 2014;40(5):520–43.
5. Blumcke I, Thom M, Aronica E, Armstrong DD, Bartolomei F, Bernasconi A, et al. International consensus classification of hippocampal sclerosis in temporal lobe epilepsy: a Task Force report from the ILAE Commission on Diagnostic Methods. Epilepsia. 2013;54(7):1315–29.
6. de Tisi J, Bell GS, Peacock JL, McEvoy AW, Harkness WF, Sander JW, et al. The long-term outcome of adult epilepsy surgery, patterns of seizure remission, and relapse: a cohort study. Lancet. 2011;378(9800):1388–95.
7. Cockerell OC, Johnson AL, Sander JW, Hart YM, Goodridge DM, Shorvon SD. Mortality from epilepsy: results from a prospective population-based study. Lancet. 1994;344(8927):918–21.
8. Nashef L. Sudden unexpected death in epilepsy: terminology and definitions. Epilepsia. 1997;38(11 Suppl):S6–8.

Chapter 9
Muscle Diseases

Abstract Muscle diseases are relatively uncommon disorders and often require muscle biopsy to aid diagnosis. This chapter describes how a muscle biopsy should be taken and dealt with within the laboratory, outlining the special stains required to classify the type of muscle disease. The pathology of different types of muscle disease is described along with a detailed classification of disorders of muscle and, in genetic forms of muscle disease, the underlying genetic defects are described.

Keywords Muscle biopsy • Dystrophy • Histochemistry • Myositis • Myopathy

Primary muscle diseases are relatively uncommon and generally dealt with by neurologists or physicians with an interest in muscle disease. As part of the diagnostic work up, a muscle biopsy may be helpful in trying to confirm the nature of the muscle disease. However, it is important that the biopsy procedure is done correctly to maximise the information obtained from the biopsy, and that the specimen is examined in a specialist neuropathology or muscle pathology laboratory.

In order for the appropriate tests to be undertaken on the biopsy, and for the pathologist to interpret the findings correctly, it is essential that the clinician looking after the patient provides adequate information to the pathologist. This should include presenting symptoms and examination findings (including distribution of weakness, the presence of wasting or hypertrophy), medication history (including duration and dose of any immunosuppressive treatment), the presence or absence of a family history of neuromuscular disease, cardiac, ocular or nervous system involvement, EMG findings and creatine kinase levels. In addition, in children the age at which developmental milestones were achieved and functional level are important. MRI examination of muscle can be useful in demonstrating patterns of muscle involvement and identifying a target for biopsy.

© Springer International Publishing Switzerland 2015   119
D.A. Hilton, A.G. Shivane, *Neuropathology Simplified: A Guide for Clinicians and Neuroscientists*, DOI 10.1007/978-3-319-14605-8_9

9.1 Muscle Biopsy Technique

Prior to taking the muscle it is important that the clinician liaises with the surgeon to ensure that the correct muscle is biopsied. The laboratory should be informed of the timing of the biopsy so that they can prepare the relevant reagents that are needed to snap freeze the sample on arrival. The muscle should be clinically affected, but not so severely that the biopsy would only reveal end stage disease. The sample should be taken from the belly of the muscle, avoiding fascial and tendon insertions. Most muscle diseases affect proximal muscles and commonly sampled muscles include deltoid, quadriceps femoris, biceps brachialis, tibialis anterior and gastrocnemius. Virtually all muscle biopsies may be taken under local anaesthesia (although care must be taken not to infiltrate local anaesthetic within the muscle fascia), but younger children and some anxious adults may require sedation. General anaesthesia carries significant additional risk, and in a number of muscle disorders, has the particular risk of malignant hyperthermia.

Muscle biopsies may be undertaken using either a conchotome, or more commonly a needle (either Edwards or Bergstrom), 4–6 mm in diameter. These techniques result in a smaller sample than with an open biopsy, however, patients can normally resume normal activities almost immediately after the procedure. An open biopsy will result in a scar approximately 3 cm in length, but allows a number of samples to be taken through the same incision and generally a better sized sample. We prefer open biopsies and generally take 3 samples measuring $10 \times 5 \times 5$ mm each, along the long axis of the muscle. Open biopsies can be orientated by laboratory staff more easily than needle or conchotome samples, facilitating histological assessment. Clamping of the muscle between two sets of forceps prior to removal can be undertaken with an open procedure to reduce contraction artefact in samples used for electron microscopy. However, we have not found that clamping is necessary, and contraction artefact can be minimised by careful laboratory handling of the sample.

9.2 Laboratory Preparation

Muscle biopsies should be handled in a specialist neuropathology/muscle pathology laboratory. Ideally the sample should be received in the laboratory within 20 min of removal, but if necessary (e.g. transfer between hospitals) samples can be transported in a chamber kept moist with normal saline, and chilled by ice (not in direct contact with the muscle sample), for up to 2 hr. Although glycogen is rapidly depleted, most of the other stains and histochemical preparations are retained reasonably well. Once in the laboratory, the sample needs to be orientated correctly in order to allow a transverse section across the long axes of the fibres and it is frozen in isopentane which has been cooled in liquid nitrogen to −160 °C. Once frozen, sections can be cut within a cryostat for routine staining (Table 9.1), histochemical preparations demonstrating muscle enzyme activity (Table 9.2) and immunohistochemistry to detect specific proteins in tissue (Table 9.3). A small amount of tissue

Table 9.1 Histological stains

Haematoxylin and eosin (H&E)	General pathological reactions such as fibre necrosis, regeneration, hypertrophy, atrophy, inflammation and vasculitis.
Periodic acid Schiff (PAS)	Demonstrates glycogen, which accumulates in glycogen storage diseases, steroid myopathy, hypothyroid myopathy.
Oil-red-O or Sudan black	Demonstrates neutral lipids, which accumulate in lipid disorders, alcoholic myopathy and steroid myopathy.
van Gieson (VG)	Demonstrates collagen which increases in many chronic muscle disorders, particularly the muscular dystrophies.
Gomori-trichrome	Muscle fibres appear green, mitochondria and some cytoplasmic bodies (e.g. nemaline rods) appear red. 'Ragged-red' fibres are seen in mitochondrial myopathies (Fig. 9.1).
Congo-red	Demonstrates amyloid. Modified version is helpful in identifying inclusions of inclusion body myositis.

Table 9.2 Histochemical preparations

Myosin adenosine triphosphatase (ATPase)	Demonstrates different fibre types by varying the pH of reaction. At acid pH type 1 fibres are reactive, and in alkaline pH type 2 fibres are reactive. Type 2 fibres can be further distinguished into 2a and 2b in acid pH (Fig. 9.2a). In some muscle disorders only one fibre type may be affected, and groups of each fibre type indicates reinnervation following denervation (Fig. 9.2b).
Reduced nicotinamide adenine dinucleotide tetrazolium reductase (NADH-TR)	An oxidative enzyme present on the sarcoplasmic reticulum and within mitochondria. Useful as a sensitive marker of internal fibre architecture which is disrupted in many myopathies. Also highlights tubular aggregates and, in denervation, the atrophic fibres stain darkly and may develop a targetoid appearance (Fig. 9.3).
Succinate dehydrogenase (SDH)	An oxidative enzyme specific to mitochondria. Useful as an indicator of mitochondrial numbers which may accumulate (or rarely be depleted) in mitochondrial disorders.
Cytochrome oxidase (COX)	Oxidative enzyme present within mitochondria, partly encoded by mitochondrial DNA. Segments of muscle fibres are deficient of COX in mitochondrial disorders, and to a lesser extent in aging. Preparation may be combined with SDH (Fig. 9.4).
Myophosphorylase	Glycolytic enzyme which is absent within muscle fibres in McArdle's disease (Fig. 9.5).
Myoadenylate deaminase	Enzyme that is deficient in myoadenylate deaminase deficiency.
Phosphofructokinase	Glycolytic enzyme absent in type VII glycogenosis.
Acid phosphatase	Lysosomal enzyme that accumulates in lysosomal storage disorders, vacuolar myopathies and acid maltase deficiency.

should be fixed in glutaraldehyde for electron microscopy and some tissue kept frozen to allow further analysis of the sample, for example Western blot, DNA analysis or enzyme assays. Formalin fixed paraffin sections are of limited value, but may be helpful in the diagnosis of vasculitis.

Table 9.3 Antibodies used for immunohistochemistry

Human leucocyte antigen class 1 (HLA-1)	Increased sarcolemmal and sarcoplasmic expression in inflammatory disorders of the muscle, including in areas of the biopsy distant from inflammatory cells.
p62 (sequestosome-1)	Useful in identifying inclusions within muscle fibres, including those seen in myofibrillar myopathies and inclusion body myositis.
Membrane attack complex (complement C5b-9)	Increased capillary expression in dermatomyositis and anti-synthetase myositis. Perimysial and fascial expression may also be seen.
CD3 and CD20	Useful in identifying T and B lymphocytes respectively in the assessment of inflammatory muscle disease
Dystrophin	Deficient in dystrophin-related muscular dystrophies
Sarcoglycans	Deficient in LGMD 2C-2F
Dysferlin	Deficient in LGMD 2B/Miyoshi myopathy
Caveolin-3	Deficient in LGMD 1a, rippling muscle disease and hyperCKemia
Laminin alpha 2 or merosin	Deficient in merosin deficient congenital muscular dystrophy
Collagen type VI	Deficient in Ullrich congenital muscular dystrophy
Emerin	Deficient in X-linked Emery Dreifuss muscular dystrophy
SERCA1	Deficient in Brody's disease
Myotilin and desmin	Accumulate in myofibrillar myopathies
Telethonin	Deficient in LGMD 2G
Plectin	Deficient in LGMD 2Q
Lysosome-associated membrane protein, LAMP-2	Deficient in Danon's disease
Actin	Accumulates in nemaline rods

There are a number of additional glycolytic enzymes (e.g. Phosphorylase B-kinase, phosphoglycerate kinase, phosphoglycerate mutase and lactate dehydrogenase) which may be assessed biochemically in muscle.

The sample fixed in glutaraldehyde for electron microscopy, is post fixed in osmium tetroxide, and then processed into resin prior to being stained with uranyl acetate and lead citrate. This allows fine ultrastructural examination of the muscle fibre internal architecture and visualisation of myofibrils, mitochondria and other internal structures. Ultrastructural examination is important in the diagnosis of a number of muscle disorders where there are characteristic structural abnormalities e.g. congenital myopathies, mitochondrial myopathies, inclusion body myositis.

9.3   Normal Structure of Muscle

Some basic muscle histology is covered in Chap. 1. Muscle fibres are syncytia formed by the fusion of foetal myoblasts, and are arranged into groups or fascicles surrounded by a fine layer of collagen (the perimysium). Muscle fibres may extend

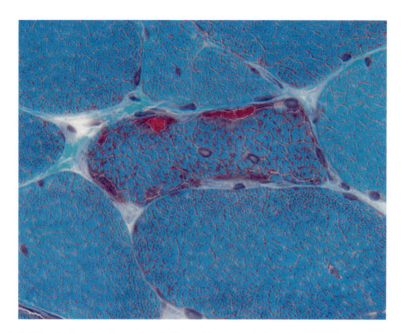

Fig. 9.1 Muscle showing '*ragged-red*' fibre with accumulation of *red* staining mitochondria. Gomori-trichrome preparation. These are characteristic of mitochondrial disorders, but may occasionally be seen in normal aging and chronic myopathies such as IBM

for several centimetres in length and in transverse section have a hexagonal outline, usually with 4–6 subsarcolemmal nuclei visible in each histological section (see Chap. 1). Muscle fibre diameters (minimum Ferets) range from 40 to 80 μm in adult males and 30 to 70 μm in adult females, but are smaller in infants and children. In adults, muscle fibres can be divided into three major groups; type 1 fibres – slow twitch oxidative, type 2a – fast twitch oxidative and type 2b fibres – fast twitch glycolytic. These fibre types can be distinguished most easily using the ATPase preparations at different pHs (see above) or by immunohistochemistry using antibodies to slow and fast myosin or SERCA 1 and 2. Glycolytic fibres contain more glycogen and glycolytic enzymes, whereas oxidative fibres rely more on lipid, oxidative enzymes and contain relatively more mitochondria. The fibres are arranged into groups innervated by a motor neuron (motor unit), which may range in size from a handful of fibres in an extraocular muscle, to several hundred fibres in a limb muscle. All fibres from each individual motor neuron are of the same fibre type, however, they are randomly intermingled during muscle development producing a 'checkerboard' pattern on ATPase preparations (see Chap. 1). The proportions of different fibre types varies considerably between different muscles depending on the function of the muscle, and also between the deep and superficial aspects of the muscle. Therefore, interpretation of changes in muscle fibre type distribution requires a knowledge of the normal range for that particular muscle. In the superficial parts quadriceps femoris, there are approximately equal numbers of type 1, type 2a and type 2b fibres. Muscle spindles are sensory receptors that consist of specialised intrafusal muscle fibres within a fibrous capsule and measure fibre tension and length.

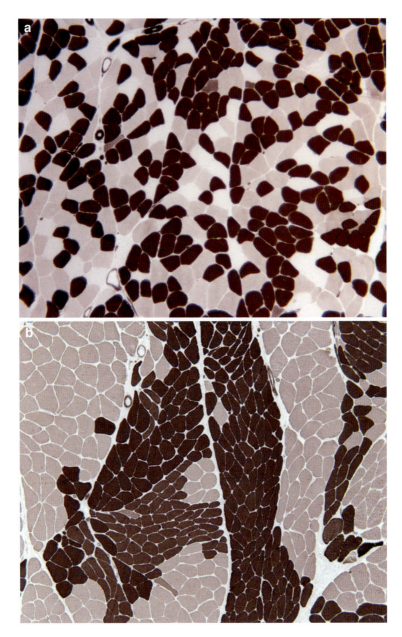

Fig. 9.2 (a) Random 'checker board' pattern of type 1, 2a and 2b fibres in normal muscle. (b) Muscle showing groups of both type 1 and type 2 fibres, which is pathognomonic of reinnervation following denervation. ATPase histochemistry

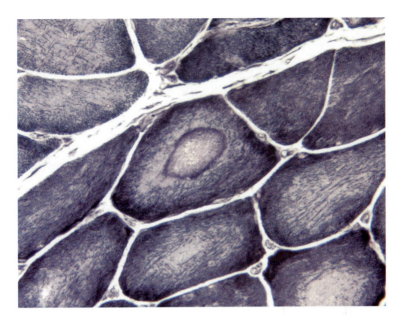

Fig. 9.3 Muscle fibre showing central 'bulls eye' appearance (target fibre) characteristic of denervation. NADH histochemistry

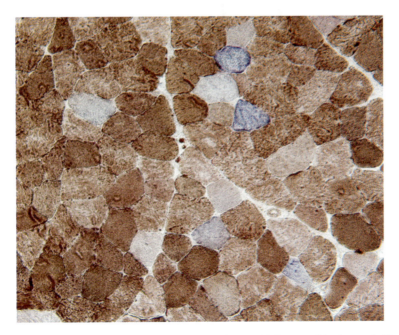

Fig. 9.4 Cytochrome oxidase-negative/SDH-positive fibres, which appear *blue* in muscle biopsy. These are a sensitive marker of mitochondrial disorders, but may also be seen in smaller numbers in normal aging and chronic myopathies, such as IBM. COX/SDH histochemistry

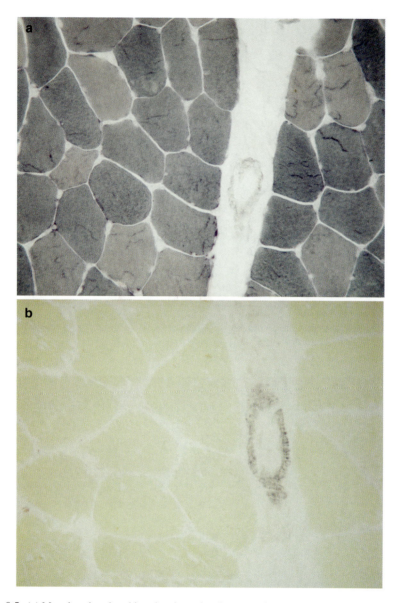

Fig. 9.5 (**a**) Myophosphorylase histochemistry showing normal enzyme activity in muscle fibres. (**b**) Absent enzyme activity in skeletal muscle fibres (but not smooth muscle of blood vessels) in McArdle's disease

9.4   General Pathological Reactions

Muscle may show neurogenic or myopathic types of pathological change, and in some cases both may be present. Following denervation the most striking finding is that of fibre atrophy (Fig. 9.6), often with flattened, angular, atrophic fibres

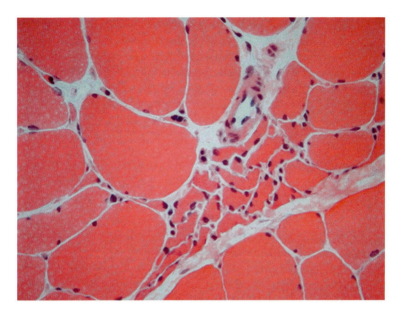

Fig. 9.6 Chronic denervation showing scattered angular atrophic fibres and central group of atrophic fibres. H&E stain

eventually resulting in small clusters of nuclei with little visible cytoplasm (pyknotic nuclear clumps). Occasional necrotic and regenerating fibres may also be seen in muscles showing neurogenic atrophy, and a helpful finding is the presence of darkly stained atrophic fibres with an NADH-TR preparation and, less commonly, fibres having a target appearance (Fig. 9.3). In cases where there is reinnervation, areas composed of groups of each fibre type (fibre type grouping) may be seen along with grouped atrophy (Fig. 9.2). In slowly progressive chronic denervating conditions secondary myopathic change may occur, which in some cases may resemble a muscular dystrophy.

General features of a myopathic disorder include an increase in variation of fibre size, increased numbers of internal nuclei, fibre necrosis, regeneration and fibroadipose replacement of muscle (Fig. 9.7). In certain chronic muscular disorders, particularly muscular dystrophies, fibre hypertrophy associated with splitting is seen. Type 1 fibre predominance and atrophy may be seen in congenital myopathies. Other general chronic myopathic changes include disordered fibre architecture including whorled, lobulated and ring fibres. Inflammatory cell infiltrates are a feature of myositis, but may also be prominent in some cases of muscular dystrophy.

Most muscle diseases can be divided into the following groups: muscular dystrophies, congenital myopathies, myofibrillar myopathies, metabolic myopathies, channelopathies, inflammatory myopathies and toxic/drug induced myopathies. However, this classification is being challenged by the recent expansion of genetic changes associated with muscle disease, as there is significant overlap between these groups, with several gene defects resulting in different clinical disorders and *vice versa*.

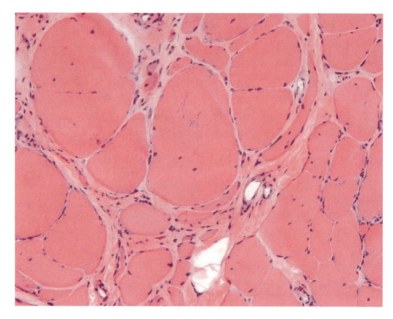

Fig. 9.7 Muscle biopsy showing chronic myopathic change with marked fibre hypertrophy and atrophy, increased numbers of fibres with central nuclei and increased connective tissue between fibres H&E stain

9.5   Muscular Dystrophies

The muscular dystrophies are inherited disorders which predominantly affect skeletal muscle, that are usually progressive and diagnosed in childhood or early adult life. Many affect proximal muscle groups, but some have a more restrictive pattern of muscle involvement. Some muscular dystrophies also affect cardiac muscle and the central nervous system. In most patients the serum creatine kinase is markedly elevated.

9.5.1   Dystrophin-Related Muscular Dystrophies

These are Xp21-linked disorders (Table 9.4) presenting in young males, with severe proximal weakness (Duchenne) or milder features (Becker). New mutations are rare in Becker, but seen in about 30 % cases of Duchenne. Cardiac involvement is common and some mutations present as an isolated cardiomyopathy. Female carriers may be symptomatic, and rare cases of severe disease in girls have been associated with autosomal translocation of the dystrophin gene.

Table 9.4 Dystrophin-related disorders

Condition	Gene defect	Clinical features	Pathological features
Duchenne muscular dystrophy	*Dystrophin* (often 'frame shift')	Delayed motor milestones, proximal weakness, contractures, waddling gait, lumbar lordosis, difficulty in rising from floor (Gower's sign), calf hypertrophy, intellectual impairment in approximately a third, cardiac involvement common, wheelchair bound in teens.	Severe dystrophic changes with extensive fibrosis, fibre necrosis and usually absent dystrophin expression.
Becker muscular dystrophy	*Dystrophin* (usually 'in frame')	As above, but milder, cramps on exercise more common, intellectual impairment uncommon.	Milder myopathic changes, dystrophin protein expression – usually reduced but not absent.
Female carriers	*Dystrophin*	Most asymptomatic, but some have cramps or calf hypertrophy. Many have raised creatine kinase.	May have mild myopathic changes. Mosaic pattern of dystrophin loss (Fig. 9.8).

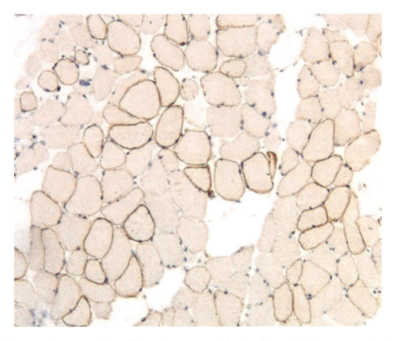

Fig. 9.8 Mosaic pattern of membrane immunoreactivity for dystrophin in symptomatic female carrier of Duchenne muscular dystrophy. Immunohistochemistry for dystrophin

9.5.2   Limb Girdle Muscular Dystrophies

These are a group of inherited disorders (Table 9.5) presenting in childhood or early adult life with progressive limb girdle weakness and are usually autosomal recessive (LGMD1), but sometimes dominant (LGMD2). Most cases have a mildly elevated creatine kinase. In some cases the weakness may be severe, but in many ambulation is maintained into adult life. The pathological features include chronic myopathic change with necrosis, and in some cases prominent lobulated fibres. Loss of expression of the relevant proteins can be detected in many.

Table 9.5 Limb girdle muscular dystrophies

Disease name	Gene defect	Clinical features	Pathological features
LGMD1A	*Myotilin*	Calf wasting. Overlap with myofibrillar myopathy.	Nemaline rods may be present.
LGMD1B	*Lamin-A/C*	Overlap with Emery Dreifuss dystrophy. Cardiac conduction defect.	May have vacuoles and inclusions.
LGMD1C	*Caveolin-3*	Rippling muscle disease, distal myopathy, hyperCKemia, proximal myopathy, exercise induced cramps, muscle hypertrophy.	Reduced caveolin-3 expression in muscle.
LGMD1D	*Desmin*	Overlap with myofibrillar myopathy. Proximal myopathy, cardiomyopathy.	Vacuoles and inclusions in muscle fibres.
LGMD1E	*DNAJB6/heat shock protein 40*	May have distal weakness and dysphagia.	Vacuoles and cytoplasmic bodies.
LGMD1F-H	Unknown	Proximal weakness, may have contractures and calf hypertrophy.	May have vacuoles and inclusions.
LGMD2A	*Calpain-3*	Scapular winging, calf wasting.	Reduced calpain-3 expression in muscle.
LGMD2B/ Miyoshi	*Dysferlin*	Inability to walk on toes common.	Reduced dysferlin expression in muscle.

Table 9.5 (continued)

Disease name	Gene defect	Clinical features	Pathological features
LGMD2C	*γ – sarcoglycan*	Scapular winging, cramps on exercise.	Reduced dystrophin and sarcoglycan expression in muscle.
LGMD2D	*α – sarcoglycan*	Scapular winging, cramps on exercise.	Reduced dystrophin and sarcoglycan expression in muscle.
LGMD2E	*β – sarcoglycan*	Scapular winging, cramps on exercise, cardiomyopathy common.	Reduced dystrophin and sarcoglycan expression in muscle.
LGMD2F	*δ – sarcoglycan*	Scapular winging, cramps on exercise, cardiomyopathy common.	Reduced dystrophin and sarcoglycan expression in muscle.
LGMD2G	*Telethonin*	Proximal and distal, cardiac involvement.	Absent telethonin, may have vacuoles.
LGMD2H	*Tripartite motif containing 32 protein (TRIM 32)*	Mild proximal weakness.	Vacuoles, Z-disc streaming, dilated sarcotubules.
LGMD2I	*Fukutin-related protein (FKRP)*	Waddling gait in children, cramps on exercise, respiratory failure, cardiomyopathy common.	May have reduced α –dystroglycan.
LGMD2J	*Titin*	Distal myopathy in legs.	May have vacuoles.
LGMD2K	*Protein-O-mannosyltransferase 1 (POMT1)*	Mental retardation, proximal weakness, contractures.	
LGMD2L	*Anoctamin 5*	Inability to walk on toes. Asymmetric, quadriceps involved, muscle pain.	
LGMD2M	*Fukutin*	Hypotonia, motor delay, muscle wasting, contractures, spinal rigidity.	Reduced α –dystroglycan.
LGMD2N	*Protein-O-mannosyltransferase 2 (POMT2)*	Calf hypertrophy, scapular winging	Reduced α –dystroglycan.
LGMD2O	*Protein-O-mannose beta-1 2-n acetylglucosaminyltransferase*	Calf and quadriceps hypertrophy.	Reduced α –dystroglycan.
LGMD2P	*Dystroglycan*	Fatigue, weakness, contractures, small head, mental retardation.	Reduced α –dystroglycan.

(continued)

Table 9.5   (continued)

Disease name	Gene defect	Clinical features	Pathological features
LGMD2Q	*Plectin*	Epidermolysis bullosa simplex, ocular involvement, slow progression.	Reduced plectin. Vacuoles, desmin aggregates, cytoplasmic and nuclear rods.

Table 9.6   Genes identified in congenital muscular dystrophy

Merosin deficient congenital muscular dystrophy	*Laminin α2*
Ullrich congenital muscular dystrophy	*Collagen VI*
Integrin α7	*Integrin α7*
Fukuyama congenital muscular dystrophy	*Fukutin*
Muscle eye brain disease	*O-mannose beta- 1 2-N-acetylglucosaminyltransferase*
Walker-Warburg syndrome	*Protein O-mannose tranferase 1 and 2, isoprenoid synthase*
Congenital muscular dystrophy 1C	*Fukutin-related protein*
Congenital muscular dystrophy 1D	*LARGE gene*
Richard Spine syndrome	*Selenoprotein N 1*

9.5.3   Congenital Muscular Dystrophies

These present *in utero* or shortly after birth with hypotonia and muscle weakness. Weakness is usually marked and contractures may develop. Muscle biopsies show myopathic change, often with prominent fibre atrophy and variable amounts of fibrosis and adipose replacement of muscle. In some cases there may be involvement of the central nervous system e.g. changes in the white matter in merosin deficient congenital muscular dystrophy; lissencephaly and cerebellar cysts in muscle eye brain disease, Fukuyama congenital muscular dystrophy and Walker-Walberg syndrome. A number of different gene defects have been described (Table 9.6), some of which are allelic with LGMDs (see above).

9.5.4   Other Muscular Dystrophies

There are a number of other muscular dystrophies that do not fall into the above categories (Table 9.7).

Table 9.7 Other muscular dystrophies

Disease name	Gene defects	Clinical features	Pathological features
Emery Dreifuss dystrophy	XL – *emerin* AD – *lamin* A/C, *nesprin 1 or 2, LUMA*	Cardiac conduction defects, contractures.	Absent emerin in X-linked form.
Fascioscapulohumeral dystrophy	Deletion in chromosome arm 4q	Retinal microvascular changes, sensorineural hearing loss.	May have prominent inflammation
Myotonic dystrophy (type 1)	Trinucleotide repeat expansion in chromosome arm 19q	Myotonia, distal limb and facial weakness, cardiac and diaphragmatic involvement, type 2 diabetes, cataracts, frontal balding, gonadal atrophy.	May have prominent internal nuclei, type 1 fibre atrophy, ring fibres, fibre splitting in muscle spindles, neurofibrillary tangles in brain.
Myotonic dystrophy (type 2)	Tetranucleotide repeat expansion in chromosome arm 3q	Myotonia, proximal limb weakness. Other features less common than type 1.	Variable atrophy.
Oculopharyngeal muscular dystrophy	Trinucleotide repeat expansion in *polyadenylate binding protein nuclear 1 gene* on chromosome arm 14q	Late onset ptosis, dysphagia and proximal weakness.	Atrophic fibres containing vacuoles and intranuclear filaments.
Oculopharyngeal distal muscular dystrophy	Unknown	Late onset ptosis, dysphagia, cardiomyopathy and distal weakness.	Intranuclear tubular filaments.

9.6 Congenital Myopathies

These disorders usually present early with infantile hypotonia and muscle weakness, which is either slowly or non-progressive, although a few cases may present in adulthood (Table 9.8). They are characterised by specific pathological/structural abnormalities of the muscle, however, it should be noted that there is some pathological overlap between the different forms, as well as genetic heterogeneity. Inheritance may be recessive, dominant or X-linked, and many are caused by *de novo* mutations. Muscle weakness generally affects proximal limbs, but may involve facial, axial, ocular and diaphragmatic muscles. Arthogryposis, scoliosis and hip disorders may also be seen.

Table 9.8 Congenital myopathies

Name	Genetic defect	Clinical features	Pathological features
Central core disease	*Ryanodine receptor*	May have congenital dislocation of hips and scoliosis, cardiac involvement rare, creatine kinase normal or mildly elevated.	Rounded areas lacking oxidative enzyme activity, predominantly in type 1 fibres (Fig. 9.9). Often extend for a long distance along fibre. Cores may also be seen in other conditions
Multi-minicore myopathy	*Selenoprotein N1*	Axial weakness, scoliosis, torticollis and respiratory weakness.	Focal areas within muscle fibres, lacking oxidative enzyme activity and mitochondria, run for short distances along muscle fibre.
Nemaline myopathy	*α actin, nebulin, alpha and β tropomyosin, troponin T1, cofilin 2, or kelch 13*	May have prominent facial and axial weakness. Thin muscles. Distal weakness in some.	Rod-like structures seen with a Gomori-trichrome stain. Composed of electron dense material similar to Z lines at electron microscopy (Fig. 9.10). May also have cores.
X-linked myotubular myopathy	*Myotubularin*	Severe neonatal hypotonia, respiratory and feeding problems, may be polyhydramnios and miscarriages.	Centrally placed nuclei in muscle fibres and central accumulation of oxidative enzyme activity within fibres
Autosomal centronuclear myopathy	*Dynamin 2, amphiphysin 2, ryanodine receptor 1, myotubularin related protein*	May be late onset. Ptosis and opthalmoplegia.	Centrally placed nuclei in muscle fibres and central accumulation of oxidative enzyme activity within fibres.
Titin related congenital myopathy	*Titin*	Distal and proximal weakness, contractures, dilated cardiomyopathy.	Central nuclei.
Congenital fibre type disproportion	*α actin, selenoprotein N1, alpha tropomyosin or ryanodine receptor*	Hypotonia as infants, contractures, congenital dislocation of the hip.	Type 1 fibres at least 25 % smaller than type 2 fibres.

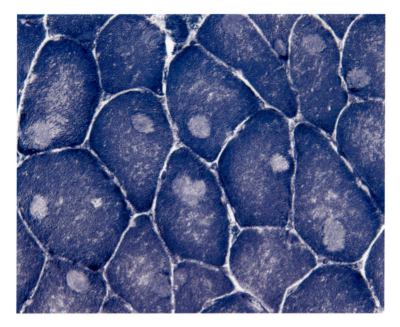

Fig. 9.9 Central core disease showing multiple punched out areas lacking enzyme activity (cores). NADH histochemistry

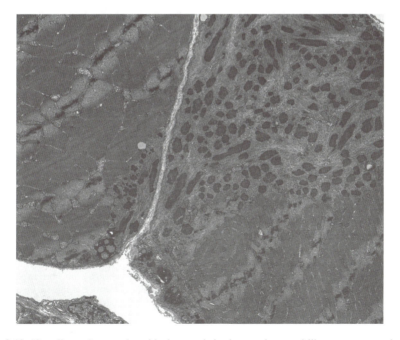

Fig. 9.10 Nemaline rod myopathy with characteristic electron dense rod-like structures at edge of fibres. Electron microscopy

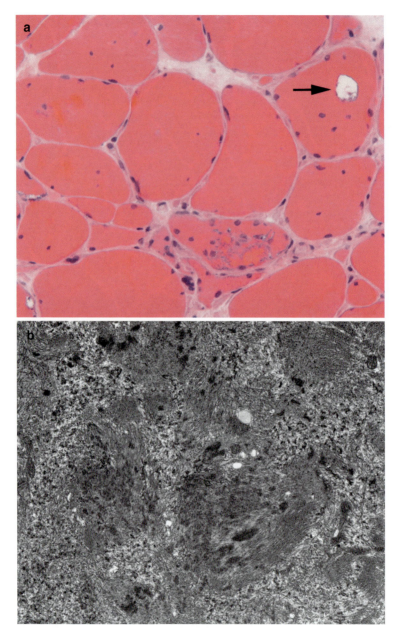

Fig. 9.11 (**a**) Myofibrillar myopathy showing marked myopathic change with fibre hypertrophy, increased central nuclei, vacuoles (*arrow*) and variation in staining intensity of muscle fibres. H&E stain. (**b**) Marked myofibrillary disorganisation is seen at the ultrastructural level. Electron microscopy

Table 9.9 Myofibrillar myopathies

Name of condition	Genetic defect	Features
Desminopathy	*Desmin*	AD inheritance. Adult onset. Cardiac involvement common.
Myotilinopathy	*Myotilin*	AD inheritance. Some cases late onset.
αβ crystallinopathy	*αβ crystallin*	AD inheritance. May be childhood onset. Cataracts common.
Zaspopathy	*ZASP*	AD inheritance. Adult onset.
Filaminopathy	*Filamin-C*	AD inheritance. Adult onset. Cardiomyopathy.
Bag3opathy	*Bag3*	AD inheritance. May be early onset with severe phenotype. Cardiomyopathy.
FHL1opathy	*FHL1*	XLD inheritance. May be early onset with severe phenotype. Reducing bodies in muscle.

9.7 Myofibrillar Myopathies

These disorders are known by a number of names, including desmin-related myopathies, desminopathies and protein surplus myopathies. Most present with slowly progressive weakness involving proximal and distal muscles, which may be asymmetric, involve axial muscles, and result in contractures. In some cases there may be cardiac involvement and an associated peripheral neuropathy. Creatine kinase is normal or mildly elevated in the majority of cases. The pathology is highly variable, but usually shows patchy chronic myopathic change, including marked fibre hypertrophy and splitting with increased numbers of central nuclei associated with cytoplasmic bodies and basophilic rimmed vacuoles (Fig. 9.11a). Ultrastructural examination shows focal areas of marked myofibrillar disorganisation (Fig. 9.11b), often involving the Z-disc with marked Z-disc streaming, cytoplasmic body formation and rods. A number of different genes have been identified (Table 9.9).

9.8 Metabolic Myopathies

These are a group of disorders, which often have a genetic basis, resulting in disordered muscle metabolism. Symptoms of muscle fatigue, myalgia and cramps are common, and they may cause episodes of acute rhabdomyolysis.

A number of **glycogen storage diseases** may affect skeletal muscle. Alpha 1,4 glucosidase (acid maltase) deficiency may present from early childhood to late adult life. A severe infantile form with cardiac, hepatic, skeletal muscle including respiratory muscles and anterior horn cell involvement may occur (Pompe's disease). Adult onset forms are milder, often with chronic myopathic features, involving respiratory muscles. Acid maltase deficiency may be diagnosed in a blood sample as a dried 'blood spot' test. Myophosphorylase deficiency (McArdles disease) and phosphofructokinase deficiency both present with cramps on exercise, myoglobinuria and a failure of a rise in lactate on ischaemic forearm testing. Patients may exhibit second wind phenomenon. Patients with phosphofructokinase deficiency

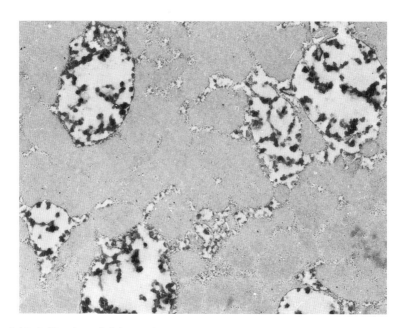

Fig. 9.12 Acid maltase deficiency, showing darkly stained glycogen granules within membrane bound lysosomes. Silver proteinate preparation at electron microscopy

also may have mild haemolytic anaemia and gall stones. Muscle biopsies from patients with glycogen storage diseases show an excess of glycogen, often in the form of vacuoles, and in the case of acid maltase deficiency the glycogen is present within lysosomes (Fig. 9.12). Histochemistry may show an excess of acid phosphatase in acid maltase deficiency, and shows an absence of myophosphorylase within skeletal muscle, in myophosphorylase deficiency (Fig. 9.5), and absence of phosphofructokinase in phosphofructokinase deficiency. Danon's disease can result in lysosomal accumulation of glycogen, but without acid phosphatase excess. Danon's disease usually presents in boys with hypertrophic cardiomyopathy, mental retardation and myopathy and is X-linked, due to deficiency of the lysosome-associated membrane protein, LAMP-2.

A number of **defects of fatty acid metabolism** may also present with muscle symptoms. Lipid is metabolised during prolonged exercise so symptoms may develop after prolonged exercise or fasting. Carnitine deficiency produces a myopathy with prominent intramuscular lipid in early childhood with hepatic involvement, cardiomyopathy and encephalopathy. Carnitine palmitoyltransferase type 2 (CPT2) deficiency presents in later childhood or in adults with cramps and/or rhabdomyolysis, and there may only be prominent lipid within muscle during symptomatic episodes. Very long chain acylcoenzyme A dehydrogenase deficiency (VLCAD) presents in a similar way to CPT2 deficiency in adults.

Muscle biopsy is a particularly helpful method for diagnosing many of the **mitochondrial disorders**, which can present with a wide range of symptoms including weakness, myalgia, cramps, ophthalmoplegia and ptosis. In Kearns-Sayre syndrome

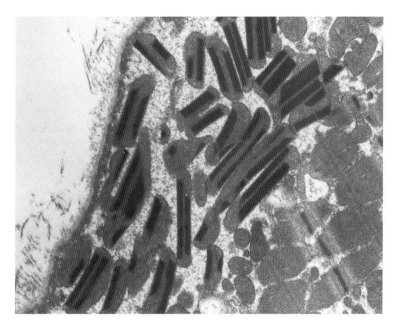

Fig. 9.13 Mitochondrial myopathy showing numerous elongate electron-dense crystalline structures within mitochondria. Electron microscopy

there may be cerebellar ataxia, cardiac conduction defects, dementia, deafness, hypoparathyroidism, diabetes mellitus and short stature. There are a number of other syndromes including myoclonic epilepsy with ragged red fibres (MERRF), mitochondrial encephalopathy with lactic acidosis and stroke like episodes (MELAS) and neuropathy, ataxia and retinitis pigmentosa (NARP), which are related to different mutations in the mitochondrial genome. Muscle biopsies show muscle fibres with deficiency of cytochrome oxidase enzyme activity (Fig. 9.4), accumulations of mitochondria ('ragged red' fibres) (Fig. 9.1) and ultrastructural abnormalities of the mitochondria, including pleomorphism and paracrystalline arrays (Fig. 9.13). In MELAS there may also be excess succinate dehydrogenase activity within intramuscular blood vessels (Fig. 9.14).

9.9 Inflammatory Muscle Disease

Inflammation may be seen in skeletal muscle secondary to other conditions, including muscular dystrophies, however, there are a range of primary inflammatory muscle disorders (myositis). These can be broadly categorised into one of three groups (Table 9.10).

A useful histological marker of inflammatory myopathies is the presence of upregulation of HLA class 1 expression in muscle fibres, as this occurs away from

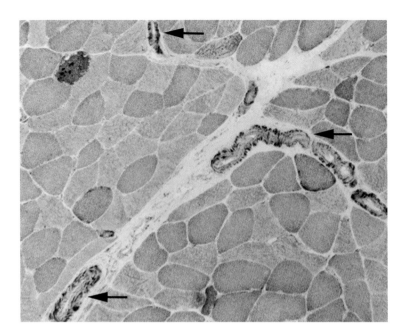

Fig. 9.14 Hyper-reactive blood vessels characteristic of MELAS (*arrows*). SDH histochemistry

Table 9.10 Inflammatory myopathies

Name	Clinical features	Pathology
Inclusion body myositis	Late onset, more common in men, often severe involvement of quadriceps and distal muscles in upper limbs. Unresponsive to steroids.	T-cell infiltration of muscle fibres, necrosis and regeneration, basophilic rimmed vacuoles, cytoplasmic inclusions composed of tubulofilamentous structures (Fig. 9.15).
Dermatomyositis	Heliotrope rash, Gottron's papules, subcutaneous calcinosis, proximal weakness, adult form may be associated with malignancy.	Muscle fibre necrosis and regeneration, inflammation often prominent around blood vessels, perifascicular atrophy, may have infarcts, complement deposition in endomysial capillaries (Fig. 9.16).
Polymyositis	Proximal weakness. Maybe associated with connective tissue disease, Raynaud's phenomenon, arthritis.	Muscle fibre necrosis and regeneration, infiltration of muscle fibres by T-lymphocytes (Fig. 9.17).

areas of inflammatory cells, so is a sensitive marker (Fig. 9.18). Polymyositis probably represents a number of separate conditions, many of which are associated with different autoantibodies and disorders. Myositis is common in patients with systemic sclerosis, but is also seen in systemic lupus erythematosus and mixed connective tis-

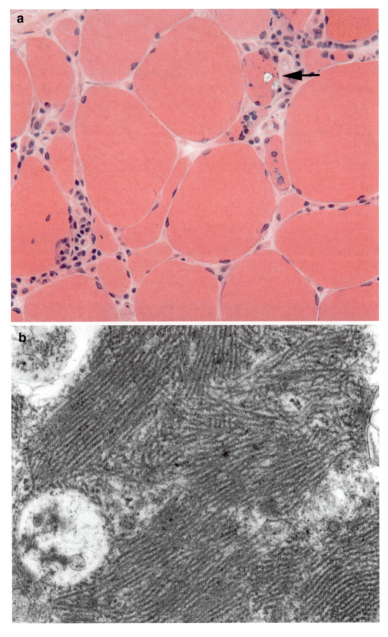

Fig. 9.15 (**a**) Inclusion body myositis showing fibres containing basophilic 'rimmed' vacuoles (*arrows*) and patchy inflammation. H&E stain. (**b**) 15 nm diameter tubulofilamentous structures Electron microscopy

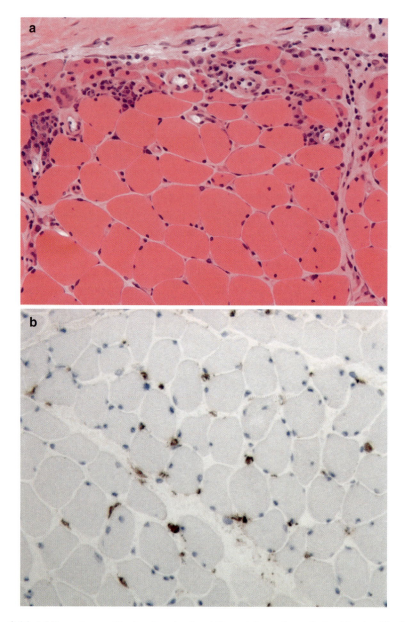

Fig. 9.16 (**a**) Dermatomyositis showing atrophy at the periphery of muscle fascicles (perifascicular atrophy), towards top of section, associated with some lymphocytic inflammation. H&E stain. (**b**) Deposition of membrane attack complex within intramuscular capillaries. Immunohistochemistry for MAC

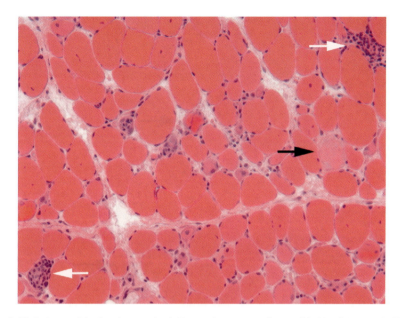

Fig. 9.17 Polymyositis showing patchy inflammation surrounding and infiltrating muscle fibres (*white arrows*) and a necrotic fibre (*black arrow*). H&E stain

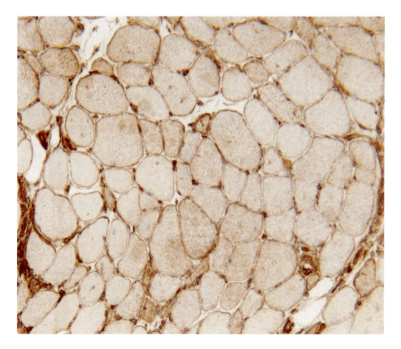

Fig. 9.18 Widespread membrane expression of HLA class 1 antigen, including away from inflammatory cells, is seen in all forms of myositis. Immunohistochemistry for HLA-1

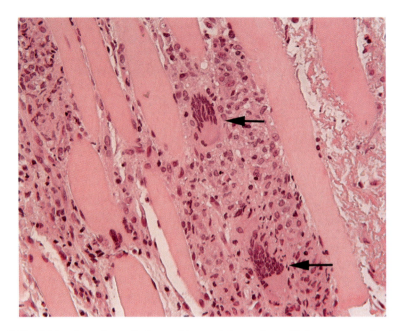

Fig. 9.19 Multinucleate giant cells (*arrows*) in muscle in a patient with thymoma-associated giant cell myositis. H&E stain

sue disease. Patients with anti-amino-acyl-tRNA synthetase antibodies (e.g. anti-Jo 1) may have interstitial lung disease, Raynauds phenomenon, arthritis and a rash. A localised form of myositis (localised myositis) may present as a focal mass in the thigh or calf. Sarcoid granulomata may also involve muscle, and a giant cell myositis may be associated with thymomas (Fig. 9.19). A myositis involving the fascia may occur in association with systemic eosinophilia (eosinophilic myositis). A number of infective organisms may also involve muscle, including an acute myositis associated with influenza A, a polymyositis-like condition seen in HIV infection and parasitic infections such as cysticercosis and trichinosis.

9.10   Toxic Myopathies

A number of drugs and toxins may result in extensive muscle fibre necrosis (rhab-domyolysis) with muscle pain, flaccid paralysis, elevated creatine kinase, myoglo-binuria and acute renal failure. Muscle biopsy may show extensive fibre necrosis and regeneration with minimal inflammation. A number of drugs and toxins may

Table 9.11 Common causes
of acute rhabdomyolysis

Drugs (e.g. statins, clofibrate)
Toxins (e.g. alcohol, venoms)
Acute polymyositis
Viral myositis (e.g. influenza A, coxsackievirus)
Crush injury (e.g. trauma, prolonged unconsciousness)
High body temperature (e.g. heatstroke, malignant hyperthermia)
Metabolic myopathies (e.g. CPT2 deficiency, myophosphorylase deficiency)
Severe exercise
Seizures

cause this, including alcohol and statins. Steroid use may result in progressive weakness with selective type 2b fibre atrophy. Penicillamine has been reported to cause an inflammatory myopathy; tryptophan may cause an **eosinophilic myofasciitis**; aluminium containing vaccines may result in **macrophagic myofasciitis** and azidothymidine may cause a mitochondrial myopathy. Patients on intensive care units may develop a **critical illness neuromyopathy** with severe weakness and poor recovery. This has been associated with non-depolarising neuromuscular blockers, steroids and sepsis. Muscle biopsies show myosin heavy chain loss.

A number of disorders may result in extensive muscle fibre necrosis, a creatine kinase level in excess of 10,000 IU/l and myoglobinuria with acute renal failure. Some conditions resulting in rhabdomyolysis are listed in Table 9.11.

9.11 Neurogenic Disorders

Muscle biopsy changes in these conditions are similar (see above), and with more slowly progressive disorders there may be more marked fibre type grouping and secondary myopathic changes, which in some cases may resemble a muscular dystrophy. However, other features such as fibre type grouping or severely atrophic denervated fibres, may be useful clues to the underlying neurogenic nature of the condition in these cases. Chronic myopathic changes may be particularly prominent in types 3 and 4 spinal muscular atrophy and may be seen in post-polio syndrome. In disorders of the neuromuscular junction, denervating features are not always seen. A wide range of neurogenic conditions may affect muscle, some of which are listed in Table 9.12.

Table 9.12 Common
neurogenic disorders

Anterior horn cell diseases
Motor neuron disease
Spinal muscular atrophy, types I-IV
Enterovirus infections, including post-polio syndrome
Primary spinal cord disorders (e.g. syringomyelia)
Nerve root disorders
Guillain-Barre syndrome
Chronic inflammatory demyelinating polyradiculoneuropathy (CIDP)
Peripheral neuropathies
Genetic and acquired neuropathies (see Chap. 10)
Disorders affecting the neuromuscular junction
Myasthenia gravis
Eaton Lambert syndrome

References

1. Up to date list of genes linked to muscle disorders can be found at: http://www.musclegenetable.fr/.
2. Useful clinicopathological database of neuromuscular disorders at the University of Washington: http://neuromuscular.wustl.edu/index.html.

Chapter 10
Peripheral Nerve Diseases

Abstract Peripheral nerve diseases are very uncommon, except in the elderly population, and in many cases the aetiology remains unknown despite investigations. In certain situations a nerve biopsy may be helpful in the investigation of patients, particularly where there is a reasonable likelihood of detecting a treatable disorder, and a skin biopsy may also help in confirming the presence of a small fibre neuropathy. The techniques for nerve biopsy and laboratory investigation are described, along with a detailed classification of peripheral neuropathies and their key pathological findings.

Keywords Peripheral neuropathy • Nerve biopsy • Skin biopsy • Small fibre neuropathy • Charcot Marie-Tooth disease

Disorders of peripheral nerves affect approximately 0.5 % of the population, although this is higher in the elderly group. Neuropathies may be caused by a wide range of different aetiological factors ranging from genetic, metabolic, toxic, infective, inflammatory and neoplastic/paraneoplastic (Table 10.1), but in many cases the pathology is not specific. Investigation of peripheral nerve disease includes a thorough clinical history, examination, family history, nerve conduction studies and blood investigations, particularly to exclude potentially treatable metabolic, toxic and nutritional causes. Generally nerve biopsy has a low diagnostic yield in slowly progressive chronic symmetric axonal neuropathies, and highest in rapidly progressive and asymmetric neuropathies. A nerve biopsy is particularly helpful in confirming peripheral nerve vasculitis, paraproteinaemic neuropathy, amyloid neuropathy (although rectal biopsy and abdominal fat biopsy should be considered first), primary neuritic leprosy, granulomatous disease such as sarcoidosis, and neoplastic infiltration. Nerve biopsy may also be helpful in supporting the clinical diagnosis in some cases of atypical chronic inflammatory demyelinating polyradiculoneuropathy (CIDP). In some storage disorders, genetic and toxic neuropathies, nerve biopsy may show characteristic changes, however, most of these conditions can be diagnosed by other means.

Table 10.1 Classification of
peripheral neuropathies

Inherited
Hereditary sensory and autonomic neuropathy (HSAN)
Hereditary motor and sensory neuropathy (HMSN)
Congenital demyelinating neuropathy
Hereditary neuropathy with liability to pressure palsies (HNPP)
Giant axonal neuropathy
Refsum's disease
Hereditary amyloidosis
Leukodystrophies
Porphyria
Metabolic
Diabetes mellitus
Vitamin deficiencies (thiamine, cobalamin, folate, vitamin E)
Uraemia
Hypothyroidism/hyperthyroidism
Acromegaly
Toxic
Alcohol
Lead
Drugs
Critical illness neuromyopathy
Inflammatory
Guillain-Barre syndrome
Chronic inflammatory demyelinating polyradiculoneuropathy (CIDP)
Vasculitis
Sarcoidosis
Idiopathic perineuritis
Infective
Leprosy
HIV infection
Lyme disease
Cytomegalovirus
Diphtheria
Neoplastic/paraneoplastic
Primary/light chain-associated amyloidosis
Paraproteinaemic neuropathy

Skin biopsies have also been recently introduced as a relatively simple technique for confirming small fibre neuropathies, which has a low morbidity and can be repeated if necessary. It may also have value in confirming a diagnosis of idiopathic Parkinson's disease [1], and if taken from glabrous skin can provide information about demyelination [2] and possibly vasculitis [3].

10.1 Nerve Biopsy Technique

Nerve biopsies can be undertaken under local anaesthesia from a variety of peripheral sites although the sural nerve and superficial peroneal nerve are the most commonly sampled. It is often helpful to take an additional sample of adjacent skeletal muscle as this does not significantly increase the morbidity and may increase the likelihood of diagnosing vasculitis, amyloid or sarcoidosis. Muscle can be taken through the same incision, to sample peroneus brevis when taking the superficial peroneal nerve, or gastrocnemius when sampling the sural nerve in the mid calf. Other nerves that are sometimes biopsied include the superficial radial nerve in pure upper limb neuropathies, and the obturator or musculocutaneous nerve in pure motor neuropathies. The nerves sampled should be clinically affected and great care must be taken during removal to avoid any pressure, stretching, kinking or cautery, as peripheral nerves are very sensitive to traumatic artefact which will limit their value for histological assessment. Samples should be rapidly transferred to the laboratory for fixation and freezing. Nerve biopsies carry a significant morbidity including permanent sensory loss in the distribution of the nerve sampled, and 30–40 % of patients will develop longstanding unpleasant sensations including dysaesthesias, paraesthesias and pain. Around 1 % of patients will develop a neuroma. As many of the neuropathies which can be detected in a nerve biopsy are patchy, 3–5 cm of nerve should be sampled to increase the likelihood of detection. A fascicular nerve biopsy will result in a smaller sample and does not appear to affect the complications [4].

10.2 Laboratory Preparation

Nerve biopsies should only be handled in specialist laboratories with suitably trained staff. It is crucial that they are fixed carefully and orientated correctly in order to maximise the information that can be obtained. Usually about half of the biopsy is fixed in formalin for paraffin histology, and subsequently stained with haematoxylin and eosin, Congo red stain (for amyloid) and Perl's preparation (for iron which is deposited around blood vessels in vasculitis). Paraffin histology is particularly useful for diagnosing vasculitis or amyloid deposition. A small disc from the tip of the biopsy is used for freezing which allows genetic testing and immunofluorescence, which can be useful for demonstrating paraprotein and complement deposition within peripheral nerves. The remainder of the tissue is fixed in glutaraldehyde, which is then used to make resin embedded sections, which are usually stained with toluidine blue, and processed for electron microscopy. This provides the most detailed histological preservation to allow assessment of fibre density and demonstration of axonal and demyelinating changes. Electron microscopy is particularly useful for examining unmyelinated fibres and can demonstrate characteristic abnormalities, including widely spaced myelin lamellae and inclusions in some cases of toxic neuropathy (e.g. amiodarone and chloroquine).

In addition the glutaraldehyde fixed material is suitable for nerve fibre teasing (manually dissecting fascicles into individual myelinated fibres) which is the most sensitive way to demonstrate demyelination and can demonstrate structures such as tomaculae, in hereditary neuropathy with liability to pressure palsies.

10.3   Normal Structure of Peripheral Nerve

The basic structure of peripheral nerve is described in Chap. 1. Myelinated nerve fibres range in size from 2 to 17 μm in diameter, but have a bimodal distribution with small diameter myelinated fibres approximately 5 μm in diameter and larger fibres around 10 μm in diameter. The proportion of small and large diameter fibres varies between nerves, as does the density. In the sural nerve the myelinated fibre density ranges from around 5,000–8,000/mm², with an age dependent decline. The thickness of the myelin sheath is proportionate to the axon diameter and the ratio of axon diameter to total nerve fibre diameter is known as the G-ratio (normally is between 0.5 and 0.7). The G-ratio may increase in demyelinating neuropathies, where there is remyelination, which results in a thinner myelin sheath than expected for the size of the axon. Each myelinated segment is associated with a Schwann cell, which produces and maintains the myelin. Within the nerve fascicle there are large numbers of unmyelinated fibres, which occur in clusters surrounded by non-myelinating Schwann cells (Remak cells), and are best seen at electron microscopy (see Chap. 1).

10.4   General Pathological Reactions

Peripheral nerves generally show two major patterns of pathology: axonal degeneration and segmental demyelination. The majority of peripheral neuropathies are characterised by an axonal pattern of degeneration, with Wallerian type distal degeneration with the formation of ovoids containing myelin and axonal debris eventually ingested by Schwann cells and macrophages. Wallerian degeneration extends proximally to the next intact node of Ranvier, from which the nerve may attempt regeneration by sprouting new axons to form a regenerating cluster (Fig. 10.1). Axonal neuropathies may also be characterised by distal dieback phenomenon, with axonal atrophy and degeneration with relatively little regeneration. Following Wallerian degeneration, the neuronal cell body may undergo chromatolysis several days later, with loss of its Nissl substance and peripheral displacement of the nucleus.

Demyelinating neuropathies are characterised by primary loss of myelin sheaths, which may show regeneration, which results in inappropriately thin myelin sheaths and short internodes. Repeated episodes of demyelination and remyelination result in the formation concentric rings resembling onion bulbs (Fig. 10.2). It should be noted that demyelinated neuropathies may eventually result in axonal loss, and in some axonal neuropathies, an element of demyelination may be seen.

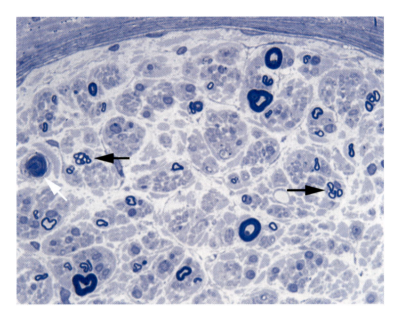

Fig. 10.1 Chronic axonal neuropathy showing scattered regenerating clusters (*black arrows*) and an occasional acutely degeneration fibre (*white arrow*). Toluidine blue stain, resin embedded section

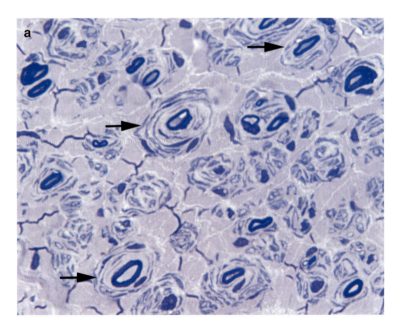

Fig. 10.2 (**a**) Chronic demyelinating neuropathy showing the formation of onion-bulbs (*arrows*). Toluidine blue stain, resin embedded section. (**b**) Onion bulb composed of concentrically arranged schwann cells surrounding a central axon, which is partly covered by thin myelin. Electron microscopy. (**c**) Fibre showing segmental demyelination. Teased fibre preparation

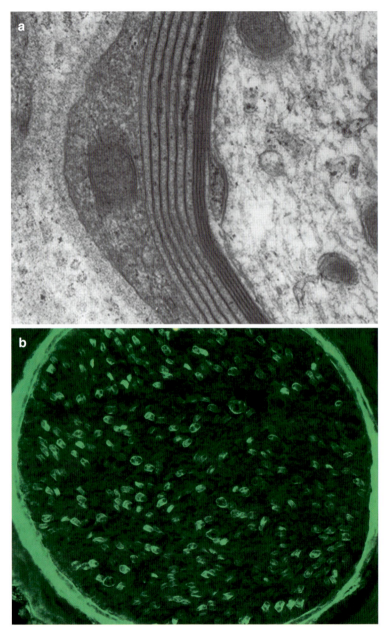

Fig. 10.4 (**a**) Anti-MAG-associated demyelinating neuropathy showing characteristic widely spaced myelin lamellae. Electron microscopy. (**b**) Deposition of IgM is seen in many of the myelin sheaths. Immunofluorescent immunohistochemistry for IgM

10.10   Amyloid Neuropathies

Amyloid deposition may occur in a large number of different disorders, however, amyloid neuropathy is generally only seen in patients with light chain associated amyloidosis and familial amyloid neuropathies, due to mutations in *transthyretin gene*, or less commonly, *gelsolin* or *apolipoprotein A genes*. Patients with light chain associated amyloidosis (primary amyloidosis) may have an isolated plasma cell tumour, multiple myeloma or Waldenstrom's macroglobulinemia. Amyloid neuropathy typically causes a painful sensory neuropathy, often with autonomic involvement. In the investigation biopsy of other tissues including abdominal fat pad, rectal mucosal and muscle should be considered, however, in some cases a combined muscle and nerve biopsy is required. The nerve shows amorphous deposits of proteinaceous material which shows amyloid staining characteristics and is composed of small tubulofilamentous structures at electron microscopy (Fig. 10.5). There is axonal loss, particularly affecting small diameter myelinated fibres and unmyelinated fibres and it may be possible to demonstrate either transthyretin or light chain by immunohistochemistry.

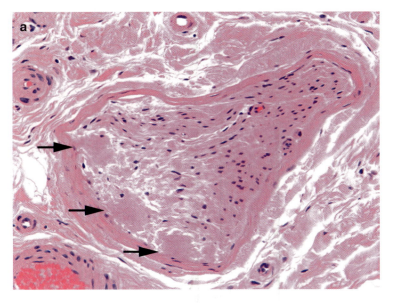

Fig. 10.5 (**a**) Amyloid neuropathy showing proteinaceous deposits of amorphous material (*arrows*) within nerve fascicles. H&E stain. (**b**) Amyloid deposits highlighted with a Congo red stain. (**c**) Tubulofilaments, approximately 8 nm diameter, characteristic of amyloid. Electron microscopy

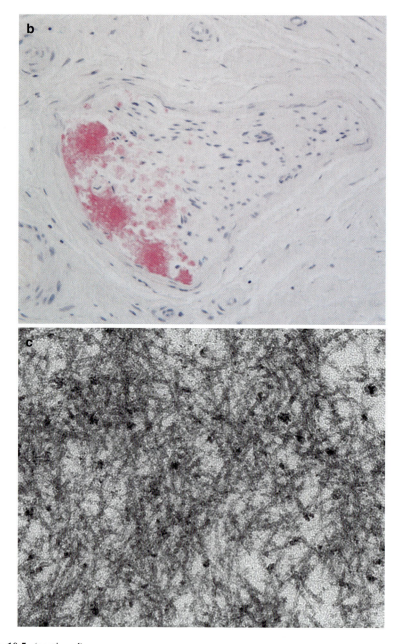

Fig. 10.5 (continued)

10.11   Miscellaneous Neuropathies

10.11.1   Paraneoplastic Neuropathy

Paraneoplastic neuropathy may occur with an underlying tumour, sometimes associated with autoantibodies, (anti-Hu and anti-CV2/CRMP5) including carcinoma and lymphoma, producing a sensorimotor axonal polyneuropathy. Histologically, there may be perivascular inflammation and loss of neurons from the sensory ganglia and posterior column degeneration in the spinal cord. In addition, there may be direct tumour infiltration of nerves, particularly in patients with non-Hodgkin's lymphoma, which may result in a painful neuropathy.

10.11.2   Critical Illness Neuromyopathy

Critical illness neuromyopathy may occur in patients on intensive care units, particularly those with severe sepsis and multi-organ failure. Nerve conduction studies suggest an axonal process.

10.11.3   Carpal Tunnel Syndrome

Carpal tunnel syndrome is common in hypothyroidism and acromegaly, however generalised demyelinating neuropathies may also be seen occasionally in these conditions.

10.12   Hereditary Neuropathies

A large number of inherited disorders may result in a neuropathy, most of which have clearly defined genetic changes and will not be discussed in detail. Some are part of a more widespread systemic disorder and others, listed below, predominantly result in a neuropathy. The classification is constantly evolving, with some neuropathies falling into more than one category, as the genetic causes are discovered. There is also interchangeable terminology such as Charcot-Marie-Tooth disease (CMT) and hereditary motor and sensory neuropathy (HMSN). In general, hereditary sensory and autonomic neuropathies (HSAN) present in infants and children with progressive distal sensory loss and prominent autonomic involvement and the CMT disorders, with slowly progressive distal sensory loss and weakness.

Table 10.2   Hereditary neuropathies (simplified)

Name, *inheritance*	Gene defects	Pathological features
CMT1 (HMSN1), *most AD*	*Peripheral myelin protein (PMP)-22 (80 %), myelin protein zero (MPZ), early growth response 2*	Chronic demyelinating hypertrophic neuropathy with prominent onion-bulb formations
CMT2 (HMSN2), *AD, AR*	*Mitochondrial fusion protein 2, RAB7, glycil tRNA synthetase (GARS), lamin A/C*	Chronic axonal neuropathy
CMTX, *XL*	*Connexin 32/gap junction protein B1*	Axonal and demyelinating
Dejerine-Sottas disease (HMSN3), *AD, AR, sporadic*	*PMP-22, MPZ*	Demyelinating neuropathy with onion-bulb formations, focally folded myelin sheaths
CMT4, *AR*	*Ganglioside induced differentiation associated protein 1 (GDAP1), SH3 domain and tetratricopeptide repeat domain 2 encoding protein (SH3TC3)*	Myelinated fibre loss and hypomyelination
HNPP (tomaculous neuropathy), *AD*	*PMP-22*	Demyelinated neuropathy with formation of tomaculae
Hereditary neuralgic amyotrophy, *AD*	Unknown	Unknown
HSAN1, *AD*	*Serine-palmitoyl transferase 1*	Loss of small diameter myelinated and unmyelinated fibres
HSAN2 (Morvan's disease), *sporadic or AR*	*Protein kinase with no lysine 1 (PRKWNL)*	Nerve hypoplasia
HSAN3 (Riley-Day syndrome), *AR*	*Inhibitor of kappa light chain polypeptide (IKBKAP)*	Loss of unmyelinated fibres
HSAN4 (congenital insensitivity to pain), *AR*	*Neurotrophin receptor tyrosine kinase 1 (NTRK1)*	Loss of small neurons in spinal ganglia and small fibres in posterior columns
HSAN5, *AR*	*Nerve growth factor beta (NGFB)*	Reduced small diameter myelinated fibres

Table 10.2 offers a simplified approach, with some of the more common gene defects listed.

There are a number of other systemic disorders that also are associated with a peripheral neuropathy including sphingolipidoses including Krabbe's disease (galactosylceramide lipidosis), metachromatic leukodystrophy, Fabry's disease, Farber disease, gangliosidoses, Niemann-Pick disease, neuronal ceroid-lipofuscinosis, Tangier disease, giant axonal neuropathy, infantile neuroaxonal dystrophy, glycogen storage diseases, porphyrias, peroxisomal disorders and mitochondrial encephalomyopathies. Many of these show characteristic patho-logical features, and readers should refer to specialised text books for information.

10.13   Skin Biopsy in Small Fibre Neuropathies

Patients who have small fibre neuropathy present with sensory symptoms such as pain, loss of pain or temperature sensation, and/or autonomic symptoms. Some of the conditions causing small fibre neuropathy are listed in the Table 10.3 below.

Patients suspected of having peripheral neuropathy initially undergo conven-tional neurophysiological tests on large nerves (nerve conduction studies) and mus-cle (electromyography) to look for any abnormality. If the neuropathy involves purely small unmyelinated fibres then the above tests may show normal findings. Skin biopsy was introduced to evaluate intraepidermal small unmyelinated fibres. Unlike whole nerve biopsy, skin biopsy is a relatively minor procedure (see below) that can be repeated, and is now the emerging standard for the diagnosis of small fibre neuropathy.

The skin biopsy is performed using a standard 3 mm punch about 10 cm above the lateral malleolus. The specimen should then be fixed in a specially prepared fixative (Paraformaldehyde-Lysine- Per iodate/PLP or Zamboni's, and not formalin) and sent to the laboratory immediately. Thick skin sections are cut and stained with a pan-axonal marker (Protein gene product 9.5 or PGP 9.5) to identify the intraepidermal nerve fibres (IENF). The sections are then evaluated using light microscope and the number of PGP9.5 positive IENF crossing the epidermal basement membrane are counted (Fig. 10.6). The IENF density (nerve fibres/mm) is then calculated and compared with normal reference values for different age groups in each gender. A IENF den-sity below 5th percentile for stated age suggests small fibre neuropathy. The pattern of innervation of adnexal structures such as sweat glands, hair folli-cles and arrector pili muscles is also studied as these may be depleted in small fibre neuropathies.

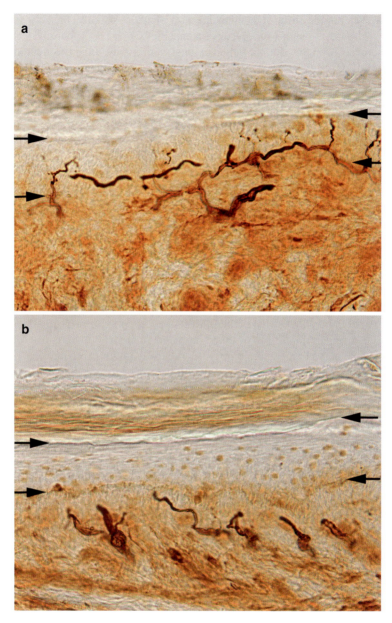

Fig. 10.6 (**a**) Skin section showing normal density of intraepidermal nerve fibres (epidermis between *arrows*). (**b**) A case of small fibre neuropathy with complete absence of nerves extending into epidermal layer. Immunohistochemistry for PGP 9.5

Table 10.3 Causes of small fibre neuropathy

Diabetes mellitus
HIV infection
Amyloidosis
Hereditary sensory and autonomic neuropathy (HSAN)
Drugs (chemotherapy, alcohol)
Immune-mediated conditions (SLE, Sjogren's syndrome)
Paraneoplastic syndrome
Post-herpetic neuralgia
Leprosy
Friedreich's ataxia
Fabry's disease
Idiopathic

References

1. Donadio V, Incensi A, Leta V, Giannoccaro MP, Scaglione C, Martinelli P, et al. Skin nerve alpha-synuclein deposits: a biomarker for idiopathic Parkinson disease. Neurology. 2014;82(15): 1362–9.
2. Doppler K, Werner C, Henneges C, Sommer C. Analysis of myelinated fibers in human skin biopsies of patients with neuropathies. J Neurol. 2012;259(9):1879–87.
3. Uceyler N, Devigili G, Toyka KV, Sommer C. Skin biopsy as an additional diagnostic tool in non-systemic vasculitic neuropathy. Acta Neuropathol. 2010;120(1):109–16.
4. Pollock M, Nukada H, Taylor P, Donaldson I, Carroll G. Comparison between fascicular and whole sural nerve biopsy. Ann Neurol. 1983;13(1):65–8.
5. French CSG. Recommendations on diagnostic strategies for chronic inflammating polyradiculoneuropathy. J Neurol Neurosurg Psychiatry. 2008;79(2):115–8.
6. Ormerod IE, Waddy HM, Kermode AG, Murray NM, Thomas PK. Involvement of the central nervous system in chronic inflammatory demyelinating polyneuropathy: a clinical, electro-physiological and magnetic resonance imaging study. J Neurol Neurosurg Psychiatry. 1990;53(9):789–93.
7. Vrancken AF, Gathier CS, Cats EA, Notermans NC, Collins MP. The additional yield of combined nerve/muscle biopsy in vasculitic neuropathy. Eur J Neurol. 2011;18(1):49–58.
8. Said G, Lacroix C. Primary and secondary vasculitic neuropathy. J Neurol. 2005;252(6): 633–41.

Chapter 11
Metabolic, Toxic and Nutritional Diseases

Abstract The functioning of nervous system can be affected by disturbances in metabolic substrates such as glucose and electrolytes, accumulation of toxic substances and deficiency of essential nutrients such as vitamins. This group of diseases are clinically important because correction of the metabolic disturbance may result in restoration of normal function. The majority of these conditions have relatively non-specific neuropathological features, but some conditions have characteristic gross and microscopic pathology. The clinically relevant conditions and those with characteristic neuropathology are discussed in detail.

Keywords Metabolic diseases • Encephalopathy • Toxins • Alcohol • Vitamins

The nervous system is biochemically very complex and quite sensitive to alterations in the internal milieu resulting from derangement in metabolites, exposure to toxins and deficiency of essential nutrients. The brain dysfunction secondary to these biochemical alterations, in most cases, results in non-specific neuropathological changes. However, there are some conditions associated with characteristic gross and microscopic changes within the nervous tissue. There may also be some regional variation or selective vulnerability of different brain regions in these diseases, partly explained by vascular patterns. This chapter discusses some of the common metabolic, toxic and nutritional diseases, some of which have characteristic neuropathology. This group of diseases are clinically important to diagnose in life because correction of the metabolic derangement may restore function.

11.1 Metabolic Diseases

11.1.1 Hypoglycaemia

The nervous tissue depends solely on a continuous supply of glucose for their energy. The stores of glucose and glycogen are very small and therefore, severe and prolonged periods of hypoglycaemia result in brain damage. The important causes for

© Springer International Publishing Switzerland 2015
D.A. Hilton, A.G. Shivane, *Neuropathology Simplified: A Guide for Clinicians and Neuroscientists*, DOI 10.1007/978-3-319-14605-8_11

hypoglycaemia include- excess of exogenous insulin/or hypoglycaemic drugs, primary hyperinsulinism due to an islet cell tumour, liver disease, adrenal insufficiency and nesidioblastosis (in neonates). The common symptoms of hypoglycaemia include headache, confusion, irritability, incoordination, and lethargy, leading to stupor and coma. The MRI may show signal changes in temporal, occipital, insular cortex, hippocampus, basal ganglia, and deep white matter, usually sparing the thalami. In acute hypoglycaemia the brain may only show congestion and mild swelling. The microscopic changes include selective neuronal degeneration from the following brain regions- hippocampus (CA1-subiculum, CA3, CA4), cerebral cortex (layers 3, 5 and 6), caudate, putamen and dentate nucleus (in infants). Unlike hypoxia-ischaemia, the Purkinje neurons in cerebellum are spared. In chronic hypoglycaemic injury the brain may show cortical thinning, atrophy of hippocampi, white matter, caudate nucleus and putamen. The histology shows laminar neuronal loss and gliosis in the cortex. Overall, the brain changes in hypoglycaemia are similar, but not identical, to those seen in hypoxic-ischaemic injury [1, 2].

11.1.2 Electrolyte Imbalance

Amongst all the different serum electrolytes, the disturbances in the sodium and calcium are the most common and cause significant morbidity.

The causes for *hyponatremia* are varied and include- excess water ingestion/ intravenous infusion of fluids, syndrome of inappropriate anti-diuretic hormone secretion (SIADH), diuretics, adrenal insufficiency, hypothyroidism, cirrhosis, renal or cardiac failure. The symptoms of hyponatremia include lethargy, headache, nausea and vomiting, leading into seizures, coma and death. The brain is swollen due to intracellular accumulation of fluid. Rapid correction of hyponatremia by infusion of hypertonic saline may result in a monophasic demyelinating condition affecting pons (central pontine myelinolysis) (Figs. 11.1 and 11.2a), and/or extra-pontine structures (extra-pontine myelinolysis, Fig. 11.2c) now termed 'osmotic demyelination syndrome' (ODS) [3].

Conditions like alcoholic liver disease, burns, SIADH, hyperemesis gravidarum and psychogenic polydipsia predispose to ODS and the incidence is high in liver transplant patients. Many cases are fatal, but partial or complete recovery is possible. The pontine lesions appear granular, soft and gray discoloured to the naked eye, but are better delineated with stains for myelin. The common extra-pontine sites include cerebellum, lateral geniculate body, internal, external and extreme capsule, subcortical white matter, basal ganglia and thalamus. The histology confirms areas of demyelination with infiltration by lipid-laden foamy macrophages, but scanty lymphocytes (Fig. 11.2b). The axons are well preserved.

Hypernatremia results from inadequate replacement or excessive loss of water especially in burns patients, diabetes insipidus, osmotic diuresis or excessive salt ingestion. Symptoms include confusion, lethargy, stupor, seizures or rarely coma. Neuropathology may show venous thrombosis and haemorrhage.

Fig. 11.1 Transverse section of mid pons from a case of central pontine myelinolysis showing an ill-defined central area of grey discolouration (*arrow*) within the basis pontis

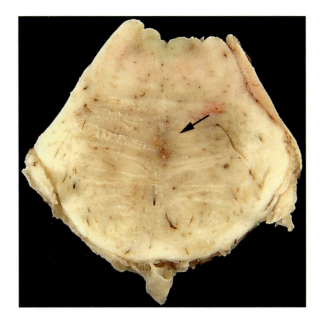

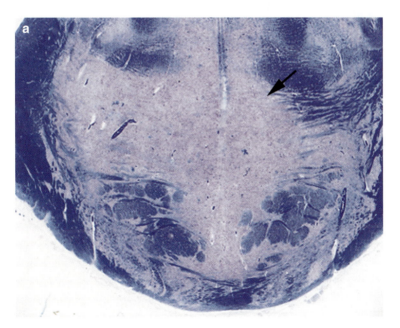

Fig. 11.2 (**a**) Histology showing a large pale area of demyelination (*arrow*) within the basis pontis, (**b**) showing a dense infiltrate of foamy macrophages, (**c**) areas of demyelination in the temporal lobe (*arrows*) (extra pontine myelinolysis). LFB/CV stain

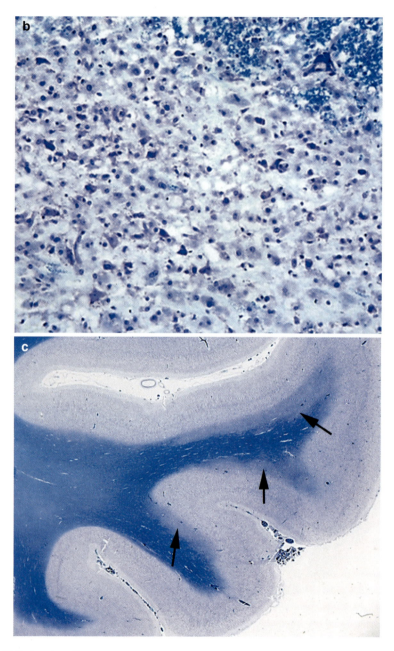

Fig. 11.2 (continued)

Disturbances in calcium metabolism include Fahr's disease (familial idio-pathic basal ganglia calcification), focal calcification in association with various infections, metabolic, endocrine and genetic disorders, and hypercalcemic encephalopathy. Fahr's disease shows autosomal dominant or recessive inheritance with onset of symptoms around 30–60 years. The calcification is much more extensive than that seen in old age and involves basal ganglia, cerebral sulci, and dentate, subthalamic and red nucleus. The calcification of the blood vessels may lead to ischaemia. Hypercalcemic encephalopathy results from primary hyperparathyroidism and cancers with extensive bone involvement. The typical symptoms include confusion, seizures, headache and visual disturbance. The imaging shows symmetrical changes in the posterior cortical and subcortical regions, termed 'posterior reversible encephalopathy syndrome' (PRES) [4]. The pathology has revealed cerebral oedema in the white matter of parietal and occipital lobes [5].

11.1.3   Hepatic Encephalopathy

Hepatic encephalopathy is an acquired condition which results from severe liver disease or porto-caval shunting. Raised levels of ammonia in blood, seen in these conditions, cause astrocytic injury. The early symptoms include inattentiveness and short-term memory loss which progress to confusion, flapping tremor (asterixis), drowsiness, stupor and coma. Patients have characteristic breath odour *(fetor hepaticus)*. The acute form can be rapidly fatal. The neuropsychiatric and motor symptoms associated with chronic or repeated episodes of encephalopathy disappear after liver transplantation. The neuropathology shows presence of abnormal astrocytes within deep cortical layers, basal ganglia, diencephalon, cerebellar dentate nucleus and brainstem. The abnormal astrocytes have enlarged, vesicular, round or lobulated nuclei with marginated chromatin and little or no cytoplasm. These are termed 'Alzheimer type II astrocytes' (see Chap. 2). Alzheimer type II astrocytes are not specific for hepatic encephalopathy and can be seen in various other acquired metabolic disorders. Chronic cases show neuronal loss, gliosis and microcavitation. Corticospinal tract degeneration may be noted within the spinal cord which results in hepatic myelopathy.

11.1.4   Wilson's Disease

Wilson's disease (also termed *'hepatolenticular degeneration'*) is an uncommon treatable disorder of copper metabolism with autosomal recessive pattern of inheritance. The disease is caused by mutation in a copper-transporting ATPase gene (*ATP7B*) encoded on chromosome 13, which is required for export of copper from the cell. The copper accumulates in the liver, brain and cornea leading to cirrhosis, neurological dysfunction and Kayser-Fleischer rings. The neurologic features include extrapyramidal movement disorder, spasticity, coarse tremor, dysarthria and dementia. Biochemical changes include low serum ceruloplasmin (copper-transporting protein), increased copper in the liver and decreased urinary excretion of copper. Macroscopic examination of brain shows shrinkage, cavitation and brown discolouration of putamen and caudate nucleus. These affected areas show neuronal loss, gliosis and pigment-laden macrophages. Alzheimer type II astrocytes and Opalski cells (small astrocytic cells with dark nuclei and intense pink cytoplasm) are common. The excess copper accumulation within the tissues is prevented by using chelating agents.

11.1.5   Uraemic Encephalopathy

Uraemic encephalopathy develops in patients with renal failure. It is believed to be caused by accumulation of toxic metabolites including urea and alterations in neurotransmitters. The symptoms range from mild cognitive changes to delirium and coma. Peripheral neuropathy is common. The neuropathology shows non-specific abnormalities which include cerebral atrophy, gliosis and foci of perivascular demyelination. Rare cases may show central pontine or extra-pontine myelinolysis. Patients with end-stage renal disease on dialysis can present with two distinct disorders- dialysis disequilibrium syndrome (due to water intoxication) and dialysis dementia (due to aluminium toxicity).

11.1.6   Amino Acid Disorders

These are quite rare, mostly autosomal recessive disorders of amino acid metabolism presenting in neonatal life with various nonspecific symptoms and signs. There are several biochemical screening tests which help in making an early diagnosis. This is important because prompt and early treatment with dietary manipulation can prevent future irreversible brain damage. Table 11.1 highlights the salient features of common amino acid disorders.

11.1.7   Urea Cycle Disorders

This group of disorders cause hyperammonaemia as a result of failure to convert ammonia into urea. They can be divided into disorders of the enzymes of the urea cycle and disorders of the transporters or metabolites of amino acids related to the urea cycle. Ornithine transcarbamylase deficiency, an X-linked condition, is the most common disorder in this group. The neuropathological changes can vary from a normal appearing brain with Alzheimer type II astrocytic change to severe cortical and deep grey matter damage.

Table 11.1 Aminoacid disorders

Condition	Defect	Accumulated product	Neuropathology
Phenylketonuria (PKU)	Phenylalanine hydroxylase (PAH) gene	Phenylalanine	Spongiosis of white matter, gliosis and delayed myelination
Hyperglycinaemia	Glycine cleavage system (GCS)	Glycine	As above. Reduced white matter volume. Vacuolating myelinopathy
Maple syrup urine disease	Mitochondrial branched-chain alpha-ketoacid (BCKA) dehydrogenase complex	BCKA and BCAA (branched-chain amino acid) *Peculiar odour in urine*	Spongiosis and gliosis of white matter, aberrant orientation of neurons, abnormal dendrites and dendritic spines Rarely acute axonal neuropathy
Homocystinuria	Cystathionine beta-synthase deficiency (methionine pathway)	Homocystine	Thromboembolic disease with multiple cerebral infarcts

11.1.8 Porphyrias

Porphyrias are a group of disorders of haem biosynthetic pathway which result in overproduction and excretion of porphyrins. The overproduction may be within the liver or blood. Only the hepatic forms (acute intermittent porphyria and porphyria cutanea tarda) result in neurological disease which include peripheral autonomic and motor neuropathy, and psychiatric symptoms. Neuropathological changes in the brain are variable or minimal and may be related to associated hypoxia/ischaemia. The anterior horn cells of the spinal cord may show chromatolysis and there may be degeneration of spinal tracts. The peripheral nerves may show axonal neuropathy and demyelination.

11.1.9 Lysosomal and Peroxisomal Disorders

The lysosomal disorders are characterised by genetic defects involving the lysosomal enzymes or its co-factors thereby disrupting the function of lysosomes. As a result, partially digested and undigested substances accumulate as intracellular inclusions or storage bodies. Clinically, they are heterogeneous and these disorders are traditionally classified based on the nature of storage product.

Gangliosidoses result from excessive accumulation of gangliosides within the CNS and sometimes viscera. They are of two types- GM1 and GM2 gangliosidoses.

GM1 gangliosidosis mainly affects the CNS with severe infantile cases showing additional bony and visceral features. The deficient enzyme in GM1 gangliosidosis is acid beta-galactosidase. The deficient enzymes in GM2 gangliosidoses include-Hexosaminidase A (Tay-Sachs), Hexosaminidase B (Sandhoff) and GM2 activator (AB variant). The neuropathological features are similar in both subtypes, GM1 and GM2. The brain appears diffusely atrophic with dilated ventricles. The neurons within the CNS appear ballooned and contain cytoplasmic storage product variably positive with PAS and/or Luxol-fast blue. Ultrastructurally, the cytoplasm of neurons contains membranous cytoplasmic bodies.

Neuronal Ceroid Lipofuscinosis (NCL, Batten disease) is characterised by accumulation of autofluorescent ceroid lipofuscin material in the cytoplasm of neurons and other cells. There are eight genetically distinct subtypes (CLN1-8). The basic neuropathology in all subtypes includes- diffuse brain atrophy, neuronal storage and degeneration with loss of neurons and astrocytic gliosis. The storage material is positive with special stains such as PAS, LFB, Sudan black and acid phosphatase stains (see Chap. 1). Granular osmiophilic deposits (infantile NCL), curvilinear inclusions (late infantile NCL) and fingerprint-like profiles (juvenile NCL) are noted on ultrastructural examination.

Niemann-Pick disease is a lipid storage disease and is classified into two main groups: sphingomyelinase deficient (types A & B) and not sphingomyelinase deficient (types C & D). Types C & D show cholesterol esterification defect linked to chromosome 18. Types A & C have neurovisceral features whereas type B has only visceral features. Patients with Types A & C show brain atrophy and sclerotic firm white matter. Histology shows storage neurons (Fig. 11.3a) throughout the CNS including the ganglia and neural plexuses. In addition, lipid also accumulates within the macrophages and microglia which appear foamy (Niemann-Pick cells, Fig. 11.3b).

Gaucher's disease is an autosomal recessive disease caused by deficiency of glucosylceramidase and subsequent accumulation of glucocerebroside within the macrophages. There are three clinical phenotypes- I, II and III. Neurological involvement is noted only in types II and III. In all three types the visceral organs show infiltration by macrophages with wrinkled cytoplasm containing PAS positive glucocerebroside (Gaucher cells). The brain regions affected in types II and III include- deep cerebral nuclei, hypothalamus and brain stem. The storage material appears as curved or twisted tubular structures on electron microscopy.

Mucopolysaccharidoses (MPS) are a group of disorders with defects in the lysosomal glycosaminoglycan metabolism. There are seven genetically distinct subtypes and majority of them are autosomal recessive. The seven subtypes share many clinical features which include organomegaly, skeletal abnormalities, hearing loss, corneal clouding, mental retardation, cardiovascular and joint problems. The neuropathology is also generally similar and shows hydrocephalus, white matter vacuolation, accumulation of storage material within neurons (appear as clear cells), neuronal loss and gliosis. The storage material is PAS positive and show metachromasia (a colour different from that of the dye applied, e.g. pink metachromasia with toluidine blue stain or brown metachromasia with cresyl violet stain).

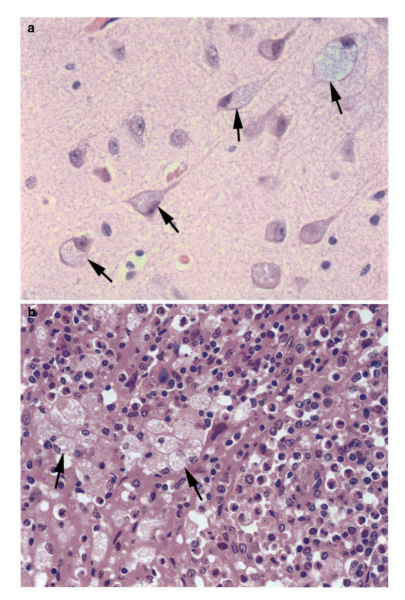

Fig. 11.3 (**a**) Accumulation of lipid storage material inside a cortical neuron (*arrows*) and, (**b**) foamy macrophages containing lipid storage material (*arrows*) within the spleen from a case of Niemann-Pick disease type C. H&E stain

Ultrastructurally, the storage material appears as 'zebra bodies'. Table 11.2 lists the various subtypes of MPS.

Fabry's disease is an X-linked recessive disease caused by deficient alpha-galactosidase enzyme and accumulation of glycosphingolipids within the vascular

Table 11.2 The different subtypes of mucopolysaccharidoses

MPS subtype	Inheritance	Abnormal/accumulated product
I (Hurler & Scheie syndromes)	AR	Dermatan sulphate, Heparan sulphate
II (Hunter)	XR	Dermatan sulphate, Heparan sulphate
III (Sanfilippo)	AR	Heparan sulphate
IV (Morquio)	AR	Keratan sulphate
VI (Maroteaux-Lamy)	AR	Dermatan sulphate
VII (Sly)	AR	Dermatan, Heparan and Chondroitin sulphates
IX	AR	Hyaluronan

endothelial and smooth muscle cells throughout the body, kidneys, heart, brain, autonomic ganglia and peripheral nerves. Clinical features include angiokeratomas of the skin, corneal changes, renal or cardiac failure, multiple strokes and painful neuropathy. The cells with storage material appear as 'mulberry or foam cells' which stain positive for PAS, Sudan black and show 'Maltese cross shape' birefringence under polarised light. Ultrastructurally, the storage material appears as membranous whorls or myeloid bodies.

Leukodystrophies are a group of metabolic diseases preferentially affecting the white matter and are characterised by deficiency or lack of myelin. Most of the leukodystrophies are progressive conditions resulting in early death. These are also termed 'dysmyelinating disorders' as there is failure to form normal myelin. The three common leukodystrophies include- metachromatic leukodystrophy, globoid cell leukodystrophy (Krabbe disease) and adrenoleukodystrophy (a peroxisomal disorder). *Metachromatic leukodystrophy* is an autosomal recessive disease caused by deficiency of arylsulphatase A and subsequent accumulation of sulphatides. This in turn results in myelin breakdown and phagocytosis by macrophages. The storage material is PAS positive and shows metachromasia. Ultrastructure reveals prismatic and tuff-stone inclusions. The brain shows extensive myelin loss, gliosis and macrophage infiltration. The peripheral nerve shows features of segmental demyelination and accumulation of metachromatic granules in Schwann cells and endoneurial macrophages. *Krabbe disease* is an autosomal recessive condition caused by deficiency of the lysosomal enzyme galactosyl ceramidase. The pathology is limited to the nervous system and is characterised by accumulation of macrophages with large cytoplasm (Globoid cells) within the white matter and around blood vessels. Tubular inclusions are noted within the globoid cells on electron microscopy. *Adrenoleukodystrophy* is an X-linked recessive disease caused by mutations in the ALD gene, with a resultant defect in the breakdown of very-long-chain fatty acids (VLCFA). VLCFA accumulate in the blood, brain and adrenal glands. Demyelination is the predominant neuropathologic finding. There is accompanying macrophage infiltration and extensive gliosis. The peripheral nerves show a demyelinating neuropathy. Other rare leukodystrophies not caused by lysosomal or peroxisomal dysfunction include Pelizaeus-Merzbacher disease (deficient or abnormal myelin protein), Canavan's disease (defective aspartoacylase activity), Alexander's disease (astrocytopathy with Rosenthal fiber accumulation) and Cockayne's disease (defective DNA repair).

11.1.10 Mitochondrial Disorders

These are a group of disorders resulting from mitochondrial respiratory chain dysfunction. The various subunits of the respiratory chain are encoded by both the mitochondrial DNA and nuclear DNA. Therefore, mutations in either the mitochondrial or nuclear genome may result in these disorders.

Mitochondrial disorders are clinically heterogeneous and involve multiple organs, but most involve skeletal muscle (see Chap. 9). In the CNS, they are characterised by widespread spongy vacuolation of the white matter (spongiform leukoencephalopathy), capillary proliferation, and some degree of neuronal loss and gliosis. The various disorders include- mitochondrial encephalopathies (Kearns-Sayre syndrome, KSS; mitochondrial encephalomyopathy with lactic acidosis and stroke-like episodes, MELAS; myoclonic epilepsy with ragged-red fibers, MERRF; Leigh disease; Leber hereditary optic neuropathy, LHON), mitochondrial DNA deletion syndromes, mitochondrial neurogastrointestinal encephalomyopathy (MNGIE), Alpers-Huttenlocher syndrome and mitochondrial peripheral neuropathies.

KSS presents with progressive external ophthalmoplegia and pigmentary retinopathy. Most cases are sporadic and progress slowly. The pathology shows spongy vacuolation in brainstem, cerebellum and cerebral white matter with calcification in the basal ganglia and thalamus. Skeletal muscle shows ragged-red fibers (see Chap. 9). MELAS is usually maternally transmitted and shows infarct-like lesions in the posterior cerebrum, cerebellum and rarely in brainstem and spinal cord. Basal ganglia calcification may be seen. The skeletal muscle shows abundant ragged-red fibers. MERRF is also maternally transmitted and involve the CNS, PNS and skeletal muscle. Leigh disease is also termed 'subacute necrotising encephalopathy'. This is a disease of early childhood and is characterised by necrotising lesions with spongy change within the grey and white matter, preferentially affecting the midline structures. The histology resembles Wernicke encephalopathy, but the mamillary bodies are spared.

11.2 Toxic Disorders

11.2.1 Ethanol

Ethanol is the most widely abused substance worldwide and can have its effects on the nervous system either directly or indirectly. Chronic alcoholism predisposes to infections, vitamin deficiencies, traumatic injuries and haemorrhagic strokes. The CNS effects of ethanol can be acute or chronic. Consumption of large quantities of ethanol can lead to sudden death from cardiorespiratory paralysis. A blood ethanol level above 450–500 mg/dL is potentially lethal. Brains from individuals dying of fatal acute intoxication show oedema, congestion and petechial haemorrhages.

The CNS effects of chronic alcoholism [6] include- cerebral white matter atrophy, cerebellar degeneration, Marchiafava-Bignami disease, Morel's laminar sclerosis, central pontine myelinolysis and foetal alcohol syndrome. The pathogenesis of *cerebellar degeneration* is unclear. Imaging is useful to detect vermis atrophy, but there is no good correlation between atrophy and severity of clinical manifestations. The crests of folia are more severely affected than the depths of sulci. Histologically, there is loss of Purkinje cells and granular neurons with associated Bergmann gliosis. The cerebellar white matter is relatively spared. *Marchiafava-Bignami disease* is a rare disorder of unknown pathogenesis seen in chronic alcoholics and also in malnourished individuals. Clinical features include altered consciousness, seizures, cognitive and gait disturbance and progressive dementia. The characteristic lesion is variable myelin loss and necrosis involving the central portions of genu and body of corpus callosum, and occasionally other white matter structures. There is infiltration by lipid-laden macrophages and the axons are relatively spared. The disease is often fatal. *Morel's laminar sclerosis* presents with alterations in consciousness and speech and is pathologically characterised by a band-like proliferation of astrocytic cells (gliosis) within the third cortical layer of the frontal and temporal cortex. *Foetal alcohol syndrome* refers to the spectrum of alcohol-induced changes in infants born to mothers who had a high alcohol intake during pregnancy. The spectrum includes growth retardation, facial anomalies, cardiac defects, joint and limb abnormalities, and mental deficiency.

Other exogenous toxins, either natural or synthetic, affecting the nervous system are numerous and include various gases, metals, liquids and solids. A number of important toxins and their neuropathological features are described in Table 11.3.

11.3   Nutritional Deficiencies

Nutritional or vitamin deficiencies are commonly seen in the developing countries and in certain groups of people within developed countries like chronic alcoholics, those with gastrointestinal disease, strict vegetarians and patients on long- term parenteral nutrition without vitamin supplements. These deficiencies can cause significant neurologic disease. It has also been shown that certain vitamin deficiencies (folate, B6 and B12) can increase the risk of developing Alzheimer's disease. Some of the common vitamin deficiencies are discussed in more detail below.

Vitamin B1 (Thiamine) deficiency causes Wernicke's encephalopathy, Korsakoff psychosis and beriberi (a distal polyneuropathy). Thiamine is involved in brain glucose metabolism and maintains adequate energy supplies. Wernicke's encephalopathy is probably due to energy deficits and presents with oculomotor abnormalities, cerebellar dysfunction and altered mental state [7]. Wernicke's encephalopathy is commonly associated with alcoholism and responds rapidly to thiamine administra-

Table 11.3 Neuropathological features of some important toxins

Toxin	CNS effects
Methanol	Blindness due to optic disc oedema and optic nerve necrosis. Global hypoxic injury. Haemorrhage within putamen and caudate nucleus
Ethylene glycol	Hypoxic brain injury. Birefringent calcium oxalate crystals around blood vessels
Phenytoin	Atrophy of cerebellar vermis and hemispheres. Diffuse cerebellar cortical degeneration on microscopy
Aluminium	Brain grossly normal. Histology may show mild cortical gliosis and increased microglial activity
Arsenic	Acute haemorrhagic leukoencephalopathy. Peripheral neuropathy
Lead	Swollen and congested brain, petechial haemorrhages, and hydrocephalus. Histology may show vascular necrosis, thrombosis and widespread gliosis. Peripheral (motor) neuropathy
Manganese	Parkinsonism, but preserved substantia nigra. Neuronal loss and gliosis in basal ganglia and subthalamic nucleus
Mercury	Atrophy of cerebellum and visual cortex. Posterior column degeneration. Neuronal heterotopia and cortical dysplasia
Thallium	Posterior column degeneration. Chromatolysis of spinal motor neurons
Tin	Vacuolation and oedema within the white matter of brain and spinal cord. Apoptosis of neurons in hippocampus, basal ganglia, entorhinal cortex and amygdala
Organophosphates	Brain grossly normal. Degeneration of distal axons in peripheral nerves and spinal cord
Carbon monoxide (Fig. 11.4)	Swollen brain with cherry-red discolouration (early change). Global cerebral hypoxia. Haemorrhage within globus pallidus; cavitation and demyelination at a later stage
Cyanide	Swollen brain. Subarachnoid and petechial haemorrhages. Pallidal and white matter necrosis
Amphetamines	Subarachnoid or parenchymal haemorrhage, cerebral arterial or venous infarcts, necrotising vasculitis
Cocaine	Subarachnoid or parenchymal haemorrhage, arterial infarcts, small vessel angiitis. Rupture of berry aneurysms
Heroin	Cerebral infarcts, global hypoxic-ischaemic brain injury, ischaemic myelopathy

tion. The development of profound retrograde and anterograde amnesia is termed 'Korsakoff psychosis', which is usually irreversible. The neuropathology of Wernicke-Korsakoff syndrome includes petechial haemorrhages in the mamillary bodies, and in regions around the third and fourth ventricle. Histologically, there is oedema, hypertrophy of vascular endothelial cells and extravasation of red cells during early stages. The mamillary bodies undergo shrinkage, spongy gliosis and brown discoloration due to haemosiderin deposition in later stages (Fig. 11.5).

Vitamin B3 (Niacin) – the deficiency causes pellagra which presents with dermatitis, diarrhoea and dementia. The prevalence of pellagra has been greatly reduced by

Fig. 11.4 Brain from a patient who died of carbon monoxide poisoning showing focal discoloured areas in the globus pallidus *(arrows)*

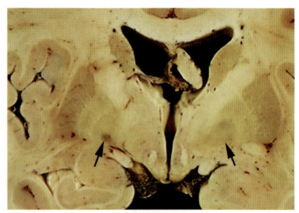

Fig. 11.5 Coronal slice of brain from a case of chronic Wernicke's encephalopathy showing brown discolouration of the mamillary bodies *(arrows)*

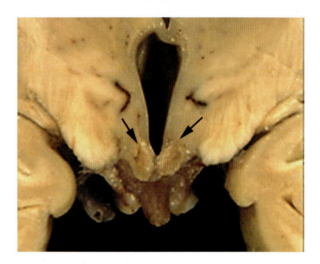

fortifying foods with niacin. The other causes of niacin deficiency include- alcoholism, Hartnup disease (disorder of amino acid transport), anti-tuberculosis drugs (isoniazid) and malabsorption syndromes. The neuropathology shows grossly normal brain and spinal cord. The large neurons in the motor cortex, brainstem and cerebellar dentate nuclei and anterior horn cells of the spinal cord show loss of Nissl substance and eccentrically placed nucleus (chromatolysis). There may also be degeneration of dorsal columns and pyramidal tracts in the spinal cord.

Vitamin B9 (folic acid) – The deficiency is due to malnutrition or malabsorption, drugs (antiepileptics) and rare inborn errors of folate metabolism. The neurologic manifestations are uncommon and are due to peripheral nerve and spinal cord involvement very similar to those seen in vitamin B12 deficiency. Folate deficiency is associated with increased incidence of neural tube defects. The neuropathology of

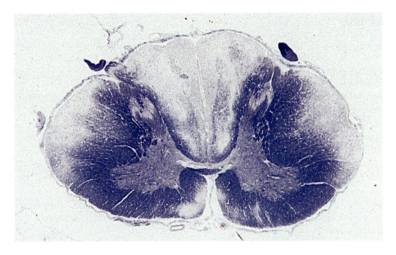

Fig. 11.6 Transverse section of cervical spinal cord showing symmetrical pale areas of posterior and lateral column degeneration from a case of vitamin B12 deficiency. LFB/CV stain

folate deficiency in the developing CNS resembles subacute combined degeneration of spinal cord seen in vitamin B12 deficiency (see below).

Vitamin B12 (cobalamin) – the deficiency is seen in various gastrointestinal diseases (autoimmune atrophic gastritis in patients with pernicious anaemia; gastric neoplasms; gastrectomy), strict vegetarians, malabsorption syndromes and infections. The deficiency commonly results in megaloblastic anaemia and subacute combined degeneration of spinal cord. The spinal cord examination reveals atrophy and discolouration of lateral and posterior columns of the cervical and thoracic segments (Fig. 11.6). The histology shows demyelination and vacuolation of white matter tracts, destruction of axons, macrophage infiltration and astrocytic gliosis. Rare cases may show demyelination in the cerebrum and peripheral nerves.

The *vitamins A, D and E* are fat soluble vitamins and their absorption depends on normal intestinal, pancreatic and biliary function. *Vitamin A* deficiency results from inadequate dietary intake and malabsorption and causes night blindness. Excess of vitamin A causes liver disease and brain swelling. *Vitamin D* is required for normal brain development and immune function. Deficiency results from low exposure to sunlight also contributed by reduced dietary intake. The deficiency can cause myopathy and may be a risk factor for psychiatric disorders, Parkinson's disease, Alzheimer's disease and multiple sclerosis [8, 9]. Excess vitamin D causes muscle weakness, hypercalcemia, headaches and irritability. *Vitamin E* is an antioxidant and its deficiency causes neurologic disease (peripheral neuropathy and spinocerebellar ataxia) and acanthocytosis. The brain and spinal cord may be grossly normal, but the histology shows swelling and degeneration of long axons in the peripheral nerves and spinal tracts.

References

1. Auer RN, Siesjo BK. Hypoglycaemia: brain neurochemistry and neuropathology. Baillieres Clin Endocrinol Metab. 1993;7(3):611–25.
2. Vannucci RC, Vannucci SJ. Hypoglycemic brain injury. Semin Neonatol. 2001;6(2):147–55.
3. Brown WD. Osmotic demyelination disorders: central pontine and extrapontine myelinolysis. Curr Opin Neurol. 2000;13(6):691–7.
4. Lamy C, Oppenheim C, Meder JF, Mas JL. Neuroimaging in posterior reversible encephalopathy syndrome. J Neuroimaging. 2004;14(2):89–96.
5. Schiff D, Lopes MB. Neuropathological correlates of reversible posterior leukoencephalopathy. Neurocrit Care. 2005;2(3):303–5.
6. Harper C. The neuropathology of alcohol-specific brain damage, or does alcohol damage the brain? J Neuropathol Exp Neurol. 1998;57(2):101–10.
7. Harper CG, Giles M, Finlay-Jones R. Clinical signs in the Wernicke-Korsakoff complex: a retrospective analysis of 131 cases diagnosed at necropsy. J Neurol Neurosurg Psychiatry. 1986;49(4):341–5.
8. McCann JC, Ames BN. Is there convincing biological or behavioral evidence linking vitamin D deficiency to brain dysfunction? FASEB J. 2008;22(4):982–1001.
9. Smolders J, Damoiseaux J, Menheere P, Hupperts R. Vitamin D as an immune modulator in multiple sclerosis, a review. J Neuroimmunol. 2008;194(1–2):7–17.

Chapter 12
Neurodegenerative Disorders

Abstract Neurodegenerative disorders have become one of the most important group of diseases in terms of disability and socioeconomic consequence to society. Our understanding of the pathogenesis of these disorders and their classification has increased dramatically in the last few years. This chapter describes the classification, pathogenesis and pathology of the different neurodegenerative disorders.

Keywords Dementia • Parkinson's disease • Cerebellar degeneration • CJD • Alzheimer's disease

Neurodegenerative diseases are characterised by progressive neuronal dysfunction and loss, often associated with accumulation of an abnormal protein within the central nervous system (CNS). Most disorders progress over a number of years and currently lack effective treatments. They can be classified in a number of different ways including via the clinical presentation (Fig. 12.1), type of protein that accumulates (Table 12.1), pathological processes and underlying genetic abnormalities.

Diagnosis during life is not always possible with certainty, and autopsy examination of the brain and spinal cord is often required. Autopsies also allow for further detailed study of the pathological processes, which in many cases may extend outside of the CNS, and have led to improved diagnostic classification e.g. frontotemporal lobar dementias.

A number of disorders are associated with accumulation of specific proteins within the CNS, often in an abnormal conformation and/or state of phosphorylation. For example hyperphosphorylated tau accumulates in the form of intraneuronal filamentous tangles (neurofibrillary tangles) in several disorders including Alzheimer's disease, frontotemporal dementia linked to chromosome 17, tangle-only dementia, progressive supranuclear palsy and corticobasal degeneration. Alpha synuclein accumulates in Parkinson's disease, dementia with Lewy bodies, some forms of autonomic failure and progressive dysphagia, some neuroaxonal dystrophies, and within glial cells in the different forms of multiple system atrophy. Transactive response DNA binding protein 43 (TDP43) accumulates in motor neuron disease and some subtypes of frontotemporal lobar dementia. Polyglutamine, coded for by

© Springer International Publishing Switzerland 2015
D.A. Hilton, A.G. Shivane, *Neuropathology Simplified: A Guide for Clinicians and Neuroscientists*, DOI 10.1007/978-3-319-14605-8_12

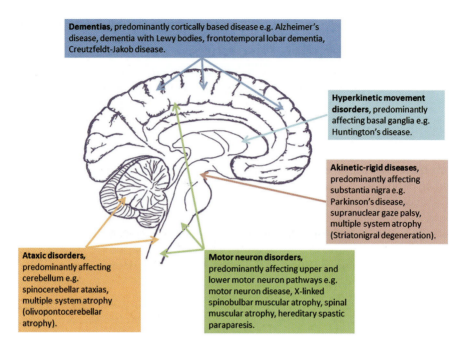

Fig. 12.1 Diagram showing neurodegenerative diseases based on their clinical presentation and area of the nervous system affected

Table 12.1 Neurodegenerative disorders associated with abnormal protein accumulation

Alzheimer's disease	Aβ and tau
Familial British dementia	ABri and tau
Progressive supranuclear palsy	Tau
Corticobasal degeneration	Tau
Tangle-only dementia	Tau
Argyrophilic grain dementia	Tau
Dementia with Lewy bodies	α synuclein
Parkinson's disease	α synuclein
Multiple system atrophy	α synuclein
Neurodegeneration with brain iron accumulation	Iron and α synuclein
Neuroferritinopathy	Ferritin
Frontotemporal dementias:	
FTLD-tau	Tau
FTLD-TDP	TDP43
FTLD-FUS	FUS
FTLD-UPS	Unknown
FTLD-ni	Unknown
Motor neuron disease (sporadic)	TDP43
Huntington's disease	Huntingtin
Creutzfeldt-Jakob disease	Prion

the nucleotides CAG, accumulates in the trinucleotide repeat expansion disorders including Huntington's disease (along with the protein huntingtin) and some forms of spinocerebellar ataxia. Prion protein (PrP) accumulates in both the sporadic and inherited forms of prion disease.

The aetiology of many of the neurodegenerative disorders is unknown and they are probably multifactorial, although genetic factors are implicated in many, either as a pre-disposing factor or in some cases specific abnormality/mutation leading to a familial form of the disorder.

12.1 Dementia

Dementia may be defined as a permanent impairment of higher mental functioning in the presence of normal consciousness, including impairment of memory and other functional domains, such as language, visual spatial skills, emotion, personality or cognition. In some forms, particularly frontotemporal lobar dementias, memory disturbance may occur late, and present with behavioural and language dysfunction. Although neurodegenerative disorders are the commonest cause of dementia, vascular, toxic, metabolic, nutritional, benign tumours and inflammatory/infective disorders can also cause dementia. In the management of patients it is particularly important that reversible causes such as obstructive hydrocephalus, vitamin deficiency, hypothyroidism, neurosyphilis and HIV encephalitis are excluded. As well as the disorders discussed in this section, many of the other neurodegenerative disorders which present with other forms of neurological dysfunction discussed later in this chapter, may also lead to dementia.

12.1.1 Alzheimer's Disease

This is the commonest cause of dementia, accounting for 70–80 % of cases. It typically presents after the age of 60 with memory disturbance progressing with dysphasia and dyspraxia. After a period of several years patients become immobile and mute. Approximately 10 % of cases are familial, although this is more common in the early onset cases which are associated with mutations in *Presenilin 1, Presenilin 2* and *β amyloid precursor protein gene (βAPP)*. Alzheimer's disease develops in virtually all patients with Down's Syndrome related to trisomy 21 by the age of 40, due to the dose effect of having three copies of the *β amyloid precursor protein gene* (which is located on chromosome 21). It should be noted that mutations in the *tau gene* do not lead to Alzheimer's disease, providing strong evidence that disorder of amyloid metabolism is of primary importance in this disorder. There are large number of genetic polymorphisms that have been linked to increase risk of Alzheimer's disease [1], but the *apolipoprotein E gene* polymorphism is best known, with individuals having the *ε4 allele* having the greatest risk and *ε2 allele*, the lowest.

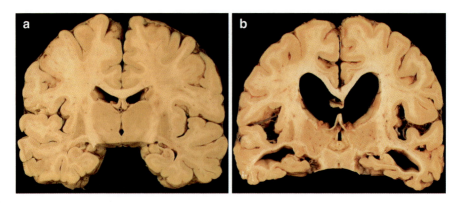

Fig. 12.2 (**a**) Coronal slice of normal brain. (**b**) Alzheimer's disease showing generalised cortical atrophy, most marked in the medial temporal lobes with enlargement of ventricles

Previous head injury is also risk factor for Alzheimer's disease, and adverse outcome from head injury is also associated with the *ε4 allele*, which has a number of effects on Aβ metabolism [2].

Pathologically the brain shows atrophy (Fig. 12.2), most marked in the medial temporal lobes, and there is relative preservation of the primary motor cortex and occipital lobes. There is accumulation of two proteins, amyloid and abnormally phosphorylated tau. Amyloid accumulates extracellularly in the form of aggregates (plaques) which are composed of the Aβ peptide, a breakdown product of βAPP. Diffuse plaques are common in normal aging, but neuritic plaques (classical senile plaques) are more closely associated with Alzheimer's disease (Fig. 12.3). In addition, Aβ also accumulates in the small arteries and arterioles within the cerebral and cerebellar cortex and leptomeninges (amyloid angiopathy) (Fig. 12.4). Hyperphosphorylated tau accumulates within neurons diffusely, and in paired helical filaments forming neurofibrillary tangles (Fig. 12.5). Tau also accumulates in the neuropil as small thread-like structures (neuropil threads) and surrounding neuritic plaques, as small bulbous swellings (dystrophic neurites). An early pathological change is loss of synapses, and other common microscopic abnormalities include loss of neurons from the cortex, granulovacuolar degeneration of the pyramidal neurons within the hippocampus and actin accumulation within hippocampal neurons (Hirano bodies).

Neuronal loss is associated with neurochemical alterations, in particular loss of neurons from the nucleus basalis of Meynert leads to marked reduction of acetylcholine in the cerebral cortex, depletion of the dorsal raphe nucleus and locus ceruleus results in reduced 5 hydroxytryptamine and noradrenaline input into the cortex respectively.

The severity of the histological changes can be classified using either the density and distribution of tangles within the brain (Braak stage – I to VI) [3, 4], or by the density of amyloid plaques (CERAD score – mild, moderate or frequent) [5]. The correlation between the severity of the pathology and of dementia is not absolute, and there are cases with moderately severe Alzheimer's disease pathology with minimal cognitive impairment [6].

Fig. 12.3 (**a**) Diffuse 'unstructured' plaque, common in normal aging. (**b**) Neuritic plaque, characteristic of Alzheimer's disease. Immunohistochemistry for A4 protein

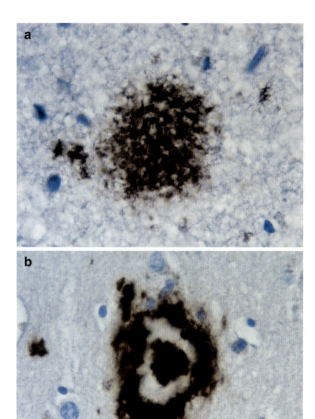

In some elderly patients (particularly women) with dementia the only pathological change may be the presence of neurofibrillary tangles and dystrophic neurites, principally in the medial temporal lobe and substantia nigra (**tangle-only dementia**).

Another condition which presents with dementia in the elderly, **argyrophilic grain dementia**, is characterised by small granular and filamentous tau deposits in the hippocampus and other medial temporal lobe structures.

12.1.2   Dementia with Lewy Bodies

This is the second commonest neurodegenerative cause of dementia, accounting for 10–20 % of cases in hospital-based series. The clinical presentation overlaps with that of Alzheimer's disease, although features such as pronounced fluctuation in symptoms, well-formed visual hallucinations, parkinsonian features and

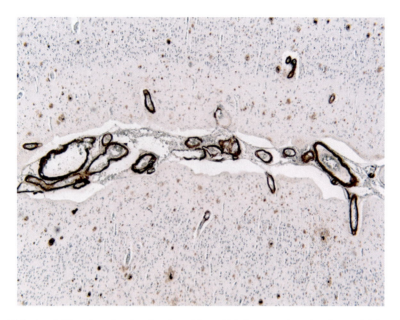

Fig. 12.4 Amyloid angiopathy, showing deposition within leptomeningeal and superficial cortical blood vessels, in a patient with Alzheimer's disease. Immunohistochemistry for A4 protein

neuroleptic sensitivity are helpful pointers. The pathology overlaps with that of Parkinson's disease and distinguishing the disorder from Parkinson's disease with dementia is based upon the presentation, with the latter being defined as dementia occurring at least a year after the presentation of a pure motor Parkinson's disease.

The brain shows atrophy, particularly in the temporal lobes and microscopically many cases have varying degrees of Alzheimer's disease type-pathology. However, in addition there are Lewy bodies (Fig. 12.6) and Lewy neurites, including within the limbic system and insular cortex. Lewy bodies and neurites are characterised by accumulation of α synuclein. Lewy body pathology may also be seen in the brain stem. In some cases there may be areas of laminar microvacuolation, resembling the spongiform changes seen in Creutzfeldt-Jakob disease. Severe involvement of the basal nucleus of Meynert leads to cholinergic deficiency, and neuronal loss from the substantia nigra leads to dopamine deficiency.

Lewy body disorders can be classified pathologically into brain stem predominant (Parkinson' disease, Lewy body dysphagia) or limbic, neocortical and amygdala predominant forms, using consensus criteria [4].

12.1.3 Frontotemporal Lobar Degeneration

Frontotemporal lobar degeneration (FTLD) accounts for 10–20 % of cases of dementia and may present as either a behavioural variant with changes in social and personal conduct, progressive non-fluent aphasia with an expressive dysphasia, or

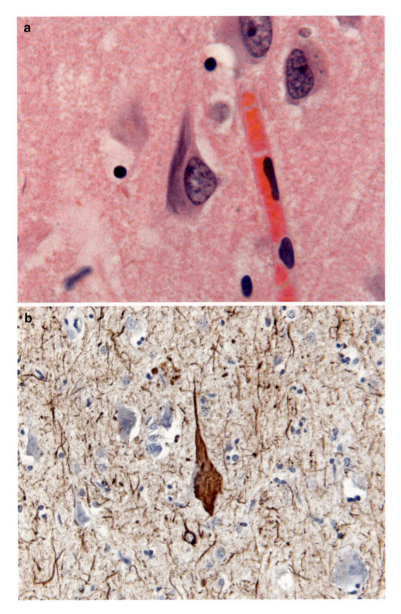

Fig. 12.5 (**a**) Neurofibrillary tangle seen as bundles of filamentous basophilic stained material in the cytoplasm of a neuron. H&E stain. (**b**) Tau deposition in neuropil as 'threads' and within neuronal tangle. Immunohistochemistry for phosphorylated tau protein

as semantic dementia with impairment of verbal and visual memory. Some patients may also have motor neuron disease or parkinsonian features. Overall about 50 % of cases of frontotemporal dementia are familial, with an autosomal dominant pattern of inheritance. These dementias may be classified according to the type of protein accumulation (Table 12.1).

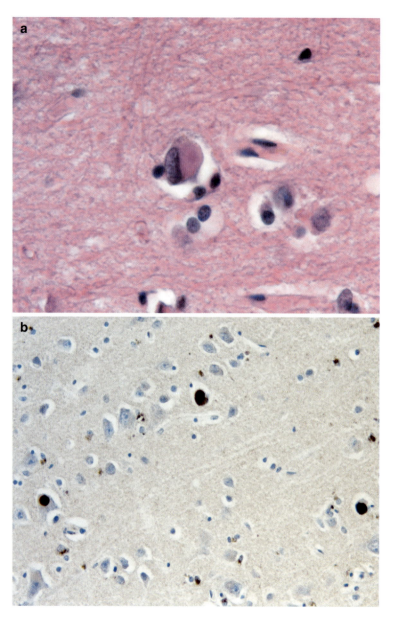

Fig. 12.6 (**a**) Cortical Lewy body seen as eosinophilic rounded structure within a cortical neuron. H&E stain. (**b**) Lewy bodies are composed of α synuclein. Immunohistochemistry for α synuclein

FTLD-tau is seen in the chromosome 17-linked dementia, associated with muta-tions in the tau gene, and in Pick's disease, which is largely sporadic, and associated with swollen neurons (Pick's cells) and rounded intracellular neuronal inclusions (Pick bodies) (Fig. 12.7), both of which are associated with tau accumulation.

FTLD-TDP is the most common subtype and is seen in cases of dementia associated with sporadic motor neuron disease and in association with mutations in *progranulin* or *valosin containing protein (VCP) genes*. Patients may have Paget's disease and inclusion body myopathy. An expansion of the hexanucleotide repeat in the *C9orf72 gene* on chromosome 9 is associated with either motor neuron disease or dementia with FTLD-TDP pathology, and is a common cause of familial FTLD. In a small number of cases of FTLD there may be accumulation of fused in sarcoma protein (FUS), ubiquitin-only immunoreactive changes (FTLD-UPS), some of which are associated with mutations in the *charged multivesicular body protein 2B (CHMP2B)*. A few cases of FTLD have no identifiable inclusions (FTLD-ni).

Other uncommon neurodegenerative disorders leading to dementia include progressive supranuclear palsy and corticobasal degeneration, which are associated with abnormal tau accumulation within the brain. **Familial British dementia** is associated with accumulation of amyloid and tau, and is due to mutations in the *integral membrane protein 2B gene.*

12.1.4 Prion Diseases

Prion diseases (also known as transmissible spongiform encephalopathies) affect both animals and humans and are characterised by progressive accumulation of abnormal prion protein within the CNS, associated with spongiform change at the microscopic level, and transmissibility. Prion diseases are endemic in sheep and goats (scrapie) and North American deer (chronic wasting disease) and caused a large epidemic of bovine spongiform encephalopathy (BSE) in cattle in the UK and Europe, from the late 1980s until the mid-1990s. Human forms of prion disease may be idiopathic, acquired or inherited (Table 12.2).

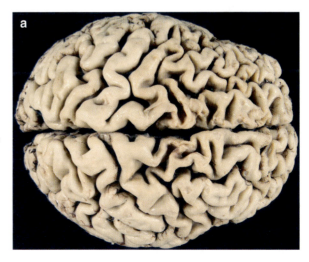

Fig. 12.7 (**a**) Pick's disease showing predominantly frontal atrophy. (**b**) Pick body seen as rounded basophilic (*black arrow*) and swollen Pick cells (*white arrows*). H&E stain. (**c**) Tau protein deposition in rounded Pick body. Immunohistochemistry for phosphorylated tau protein

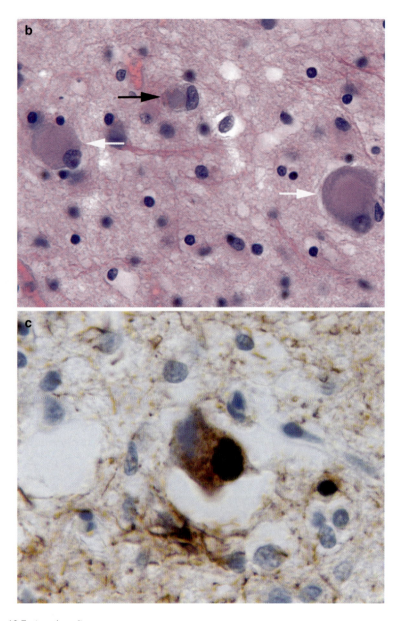

Fig. 12.7 (continued)

The cause for sporadic CJD (sCJD), which accounts for 85 % of all cases of human prion disease, is unknown. Familial forms of human prion disease are associated with over 30 different mutations in the *prion protein gene* and are dominantly inherited with a high penetrance [7].

Table 12.2 Human prion diseases

Idiopathic	Sporadic Creutzfeldt-Jakob disease
Acquired	Iatrogenic Creutzfeldt-Jakob disease
	Kuru
	Variant Creutzfeldt-Jakob disease
Inherited	Familial Creutzfeldt-Jakob disease
	Gerstmann-Straussler-Scheinker syndrome
	Familial fatal insomnia

Iatrogenic CJD (iCJD), has been associated with dura mater homografts prior to 1992, with many cases occurring in Japan, or with either human growth hormone or gonadotropin replacement (derived from pituitary glands taken post mortem) prior to 1996. These cases are caused by contamination of either the dura or hormone product, by brain tissue from patients with CJD, and the incubation periods range from 1 to 30 years.

Kuru was confined to Papua New Guinea and associated with ritualistic cannibalism, resulting in human-human transmission and causing a predominantly ataxic disorder. However, since the abolition of this practice in the late 1950s, kuru has steadily disappeared.

Variant CJD (vCJD) is largely confined to individuals who have lived in the UK, and is linked to exposure to BSE-contaminated food products. A small number of cases have been linked to blood transfusions taken from patients who later went on to develop vCJD. Recent attempts at developing a test to detect prions in blood from individuals with vCJD have shown promise [8] and may prove useful in detecting individuals who may be silent carriers of the disease [9]. vCJD affects young adults (average age 28), the EEG does not show specific abnormalities, and MRI typically shows high signal in the thalamus.

sCJD usually presents after the age of 60 with a relatively rapidly progressive dementia over a period of months, associated with myoclonus and in many cases periodic triphasic complexes on EEG and high signal within the basal ganglia on MRI. In most cases CSF 14-3-3 protein and S100 proteins are elevated. However, it is clear that there are several subtypes of sCJD with differing clinical presentations and pathology [10].

The pathology of all of these forms of CJD has similarities, with spongiform change (Fig. 12.8a) and accumulation of prion protein (PrP) within the brain. PrP may accumulate in the form of small granular deposits (synaptic patterns) (Fig. 12.8b), around vacuoles (perivacuolar) or larger amyloid plaques, the latter being a characteristic feature of vCJD. Another important and characteristic feature of vCJD is the accumulation of PrP in the peripheral lymphoreticular system (Fig. 12.8c), and this occurs many years before the onset of clinical disease, including the gut-associated lymphoid tissue such as the tonsil and appendix, lymph nodes and spleen. In cases of familial prion disease the spongiform change may be mild.

A common polymorphism in the *PrP gene* at codon 129 is an important susceptibility factor with patients who are heterozygous for methionine and valine, being

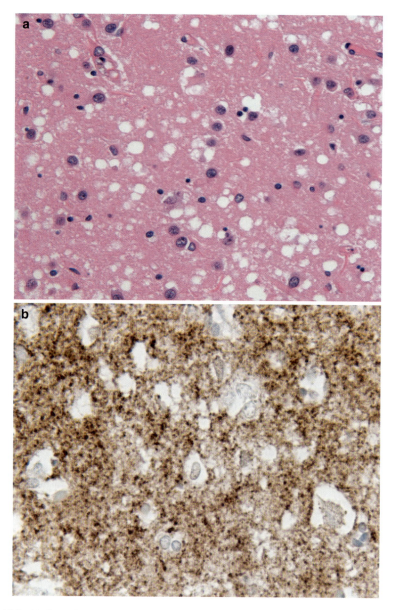

Fig. 12.8 (**a**) Creutzfeldt-Jacob disease showing characteristic microscopic vacuolation (spongiform change). H&E stain. (**b**) Granular accumulation of abnormal prion protein in brain. Immunohistochemistry for PrP. (**c**) Deposition of prion protein within the follicular dendritic cells of tonsil, which is only seen in variant CJD. Immunohistochemistry for PrP

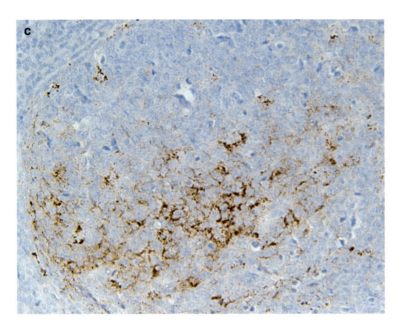

Fig. 12.8 (continued)

at a lower risk than those who are homozygous, and in the case of iCJD, heterozygotes also have a longer incubation period. Virtually all clinical cases of vCJD to date have been methionine homozygotes.

Prion proteins have been shown to be transmissible by both inoculation and ingestion. The abnormal form of PrP (which has a different conformation to the normal cellular form) has certain characteristics including resistance to degradation (including heat-induced denaturation and proteolytic digestion), facilitating its accumulation within the CNS. In addition the abnormal form of PrP has the ability to convert the normal form into itself, thereby catalysing its own production within cells. The extreme resistance of disease-associated PrP to degradation poses a potential risk to health, as standard autoclaving of surgical instruments does not completely decontaminate them. It is important that the laboratory is warned of the possibility of CJD when a brain biopsy is taken for diagnostic purposes, so that appropriate measures can be taken to minimise risk to staff.

12.2   Disorders Predominantly Affecting the Basal Ganglia

Many of these conditions also affect many other brain regions, but they often present with primarily a movement disorder, which may be hyperkinetic in nature.

12.2.1   Huntington's Disease

Huntington's disease may present in childhood (juvenile form), but more often presents in early adult life, and rarely in late adult life. Presentation is with choreiform movements or psychiatric features, but the juvenile form may have an akinetic-rigid presentation. Huntington's disease is caused by expansion of a polyglutamine repeat sequence on chromosome 4, which forms part of the gene for the protein huntingtin. Expansion of the repeat to 37 or more leads to Huntington's disease, and in general the longer the repeat, the earlier the onset and more rapid the decline. Repeats are unstable and the length may increase, particularly during spermatogenesis and oogenesis, leading to a more severe form with earlier onset in offspring of affected individuals (genetic 'anticipation'). Huntington's disease results in atrophy of the caudate nucleus, putamen and globus pallidus, and often a degree of cortical atrophy. The severity of the striatal atrophy can be graded using the Vonsattel grading scheme: 1 no visible caudate atrophy; 2 atrophy, but with a convex contour to the caudate head; 3 flattening of the caudate head; 4 concave medial contour. Histologically, there is neuronal loss and gliosis, which is associated with intranuclear aggregates of huntingtin, which like many protein aggregates in the CNS are ubiquitinated, and can be detected by immunohistochemistry using antibodies to ubiquitin and p62.

12.2.2   Neurodegeneration with Brain Iron Accumulation

Neurodegeneration with brain iron accumulation (NBIA), which overlaps with the neuroaxonal dystrophies, is a group of autosomal recessive conditions characterised by the presence of axonal swellings within the nervous system, sometimes associated with accumulation of iron and α synuclein containing Lewy bodies within the basal nuclei and other regions. Presentation is varied and may include developmental delay, dystonia, rigidity, ataxia, parkinsonian and psychiatric features. There are a number of causes, including mutations in the *pantothenate kinase gene* (NIBA1), previously Hallervorden-Spatz disease; mutations in the *phospholipase A2 group 6 gene (PLA2G6)* which may result in infantile, juvenile or adult onset disease (NIBA2), previously Seitelberger's disease. Mutations in the *ferritin light chain gene* result in the neuroferritinopathies, also known as NIBA3, are dominantly inherited and characterised by motor and behavioural disturbance, dementia, and the brain shows cavitation in the putamen and ferritin containing inclusions in neurons and glia. These inclusions are also seen in the skin and other organs in the body.

12.2.3   Neuroacanthocytosis

Neuroacanthocytosis is the term used for a range of neurodegenerative disorders, often presenting with a movement disorder, in which there is degeneration of the corpus striatum and the presence of acanthocytes in the blood.

It should be noted that other neurodegenerative disorders including corticobasal degeneration, multiple system atrophy, frontotemporal lobar dementia and dentatorubral-pallidoluysial atrophy may also present predominantly with basal ganglia degeneration and a movement disorder. These conditions are discussed further below.

12.3   Disorders Predominantly Affecting the Midbrain

These usually present with parkinsonism i.e. rigidity, bradykinesia and tremor, but some affect other brain regions and therefore may have additional clinical features.

12.3.1   Parkinson's Disease

After Alzheimer's disease, this is the next most common of the neurodegenerative disorders. It is characterised by loss of neurons from the substantia nigra and locus ceruleus and the presence of Lewy bodies, which are composed of a large number of proteins including α synuclein (Fig. 12.9). The α synuclein is phosphorylated, and also accumulates within axons (Lewy neurites). Pale bodies are less well-structured rounded aggregates within neurons which also contain α synuclein and may be precursors to Lewy bodies. Lewy bodies are seen in many other regions including the dorsal motor nucleus of the vagus, basal forebrain, cerebral cortex, spinal cord, autonomic neurons, including the enteric ganglia, where they have been seen up to 8 years prior to the onset of central motor symptoms [11]. Parkinson's disease forms part of a spectrum of disorders associated with Lewy bodies, including Parkinson's disease with dementia (dementia occurring at least a year after the onset of Parkinson's disease), dementia with Lewy

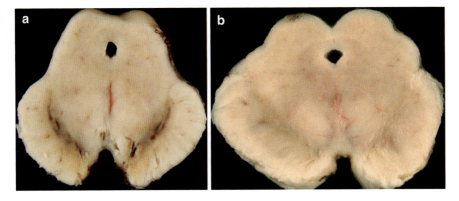

Fig. 12.9 (**a**) Normal midbrain. (**b**) Parkinson's disease showing marked pallor of substantia nigra due to loss of pigmented neurons. (**c**) Lewy body within the pigmented neuron of substantia nigra. H&E stain. (**d**) deposition of α synuclein within small autonomic nerves of bowel before the onset of neurological symptoms. Immunohistochemistry for α synuclein

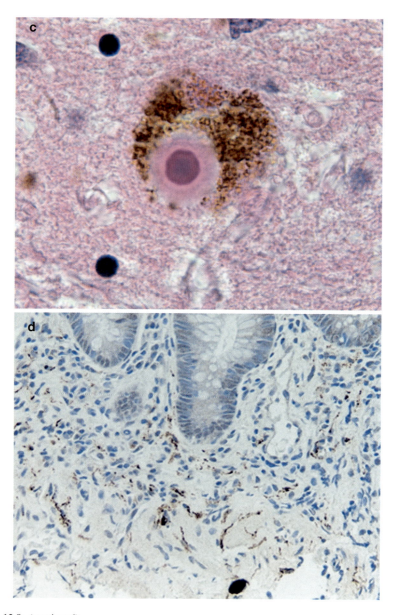

Fig. 12.9 (continued)

bodies (dementia occurs within 1 year of onset of the parkinsonian symptoms), progressive autonomic failure and Lewy body dysphagia, the latter of which are associated with pathology predominantly within the autonomic nervous system and dorsal motor nucleus of vagus respectively. There are a number of inherited forms of Parkinson's disease and parkinsonism which may be either recessive or dominant in inheritance, and some of which are associated with the presence of Lewy bodies.

12.3.2   Progressive Supranuclear Palsy

Progressive supranuclear palsy (also known as Steele Richardson Olszewski syndrome), presents with parkinsonian features associated with supranuclear gaze palsy, dysarthria, dysphasia and cognitive impairment. There is neuronal loss from the substantia nigra, locus ceruleus and globus pallidus and accumulation of tau protein. The tau may be accumulated in the form of neurofibrillary tangles within neurons, but is also seen within glia forming 'tufted' astrocytes, and the neuronal tangles often have a globose morphology (Fig. 12.10). Tau inclusions also occur within oligodendroglia, often forming coiled bodies. Severely affected areas include the substantia nigra,

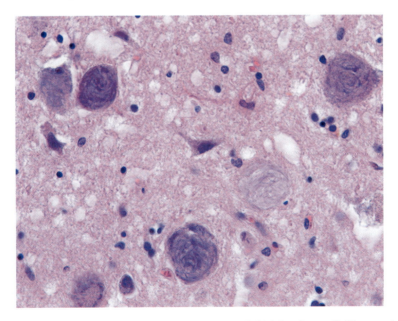

Fig. 12.10 Progressive supranuclear palsy with large rounded 'globose' neurofibrillary tangles in substantia nigra. H&E stain

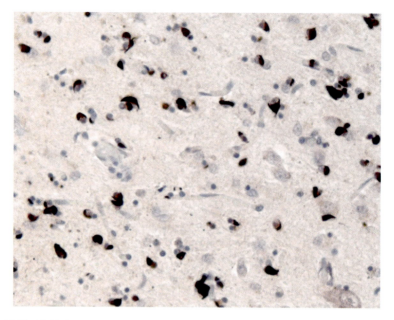

Fig. 12.11 Multiple system atrophy with numerous 'sickle-shaped'α synuclein-containing inclusions within glia. Immunohistochemistry for α synuclein

red nucleus, periaqueductal grey matter, globus pallidus, hippocampus, subthalamic nucleus and dentate nucleus of the cerebellum. It should be noted that in some cases distinction from corticobasal degeneration on pathology may be difficult.

12.3.3   Multiple System Atrophy

These patients often present in mid to late adult life with parkinsonian features, cerebellar ataxia, autonomic failure and cognitive impairment. Sudden death may result from laryngeal involvement resulting in apnoea. There are three principle patterns of presentation: (1) Olivopontocerebellar atrophy, (2) Shy Drager syndrome, (3) Striatonigral degeneration. Pathologically there may be gross atrophy of the cerebellum, pons and putamen with pallor of the substantia nigra. There is marked neuronal loss and gliosis in these regions and the disorder is characterised by an accumulation of α synuclein in glia and neurons. The most prominent feature is the presence of flame or sickle shaped inclusions within oligodendrocytes in affected regions of the CNS (Fig. 12.11), but there may also be inclusions present within neurons both in the nuclei, cytoplasm and axons. All of these inclusions show α synuclein immunoreactivity and the distribution of pathology correlates with the clinical presentation, so that in OPCA there is prominent atrophy of the brainstem and cerebellum, in Shy Drager syndrome

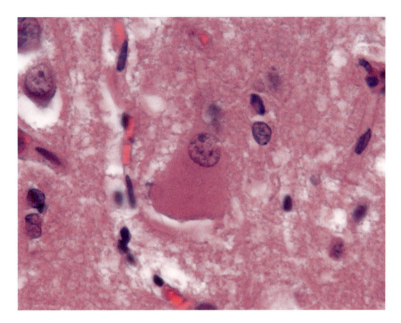

Fig. 12.12 Corticobasal degeneration with swollen 'ballooned' neuron in frontal cortex. H&E stain

there is prominent involvement of the intermediolateral column of the spinal cord, and in striatonigral degeneration there is prominent involvement of the putamen and substantia nigra.

12.3.4 Corticobasal Degeneration

This presents in mid to late adult life, often with limb stiffness and clumsiness, alien limb syndrome, apraxia and cognitive impairment. Pathologically there may be focal cortical atrophy in the frontal lobe which may be asymmetric, associated with neuronal loss, swollen ballooned neurons (Fig. 12.12) within the cortex which contain tau protein.

12.3.5 Other Disorders

Other rare causes of parkinsonism include drugs and toxins such as MPTP and neuroleptic drugs, post encephalitic parkinsonism, following encephalitis lethargica in which there are tau positive neurofibrillary tangles within the substantia nigra, Guam parkinsonism-dementia which may be associated with motor neuron disease, and chronic traumatic encephalopathy (see Chap. 13).

Table 12.3 Causes of
cerebellar degeneration

Autosomal dominant disorders
Autosomal dominant spinocerebellar ataxias (SCAD 1–36)
Dentatorubral-pallidoluysial atrophy
Episodic ataxias
Autosomal recessive disorders
Friedreich's ataxia
Cerebellar ataxia with vitamin E deficiency
Ataxia telangiectasia
Autosomal recessive spinocerebellar ataxia (SCAR 1–10)
X-linked disorders
Fragile X-associated tremor and ataxia syndrome
Mitochondrial disorders
Sporadic disorders
Multiple system atrophy
Creutzfeldt-Jakob disease
Toxic causes
Ethanol
Anti-epileptic drugs
Heavy metals
Autoimmune disease
Coeliac disease
Paraneoplastic disorders

12.4   Cerebellar Degeneration

A large number of disorders may cause cerebellar degeneration (Table 12.3) including toxic, nutritional, metabolic, autoimmune, including paraneoplastic disorders, which are discussed elsewhere. In addition, there are a number of degenerative disorders, some of which are hereditary, which may cause progressive cerebellar neuronal loss. In some of these cerebellar degenerations there may also be loss of neurons from the inferior olivary nuclei, pontine nuclei and spinocerebellar tracts.

12.5   Motor Neuron Diseases

These disorders selectively involve upper and/or lower motor neurons within the CNS causing progressive upper and/or lower motor neuron weakness.

12.5.1   Motor Neuron Disease

This is also known as amyotrophic lateral sclerosis (ALS) or Lou Gehrig's disease, with variants presenting predominantly with bulbar palsy (progressive bulbar palsy) or predominantly lower motor neuron involvement (progressive muscular atrophy).

Typically there is involvement of both upper and lower motor neurons and there is progression to death from respiratory failure or pneumonia within 5 years of onset. Around 15 % of patients develop a frontal lobe dementia. Pathologically there is loss of both upper and lower motor neurons from the CNS, associated with protein accumulation within neurons (Fig. 12.13). In the majority of cases the protein that accumulates is transactive response DNA-binding protein 43 (TDP43), which accumulates within upper and lower motor neurons, and in patients with dementia, cortical and hippocampal neurons. Approximately 10 % of cases are hereditary, the majority being dominantly inherited, caused by a number of different genetic mutations. Some of these hereditary cases have atypical pathology and, in some, there may be sensory involvement.

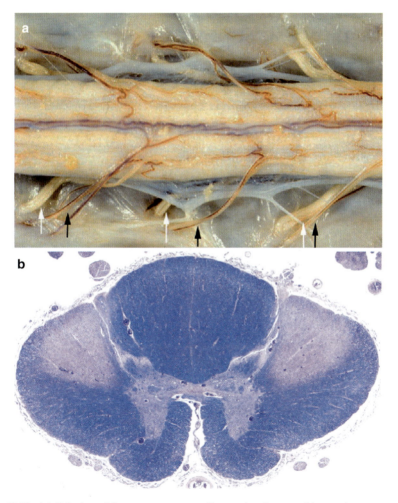

Fig. 12.13 (**a**) Spinal cord from motor neuron disease showing atrophic anterior nerve roots (*black arrows*) and well preserved posterior roots (*white arrows*). (**b**) Section of cord showing degeneration in both lateral corticospinal tracts. Myelin stain. (**c**) TDP-43 containing cytoplasmic inclusions in surviving anterior horn cells. Immunohistochemistry for TDP-43

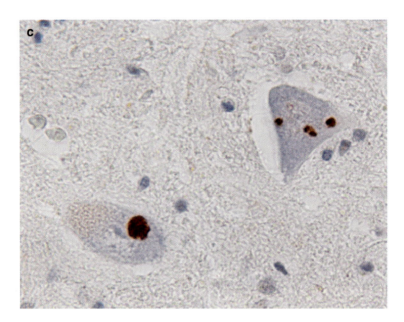

Fig. 12.13 (continued)

12.5.2   X-Linked Bulbar Spinal Muscular Atrophy (Kennedy's Disease)

This is due to CAG repeat expansion in the *androgen receptor gene* and presents in males with motor weakness and gynaecomastia.

12.5.3   Spinal Muscular Atrophy

This causes lower motor neuron weakness and the majority of cases present in childhood, and largely autosomally recessive due to deletions of the telomeric copy of the *survival motor neuron gene (SMN1)* on chromosome 5. The disease may present as an acute infantile form which may present with neonatal hypotonia and severe proximal weakness involving respiratory muscles (SMA1 or Werdnig-Hoffmann disease), a more slowly progressive chronic childhood form with proximal limb weakness after the age of 2 years (SMA3 or Kugelberg Welander disease) or an intermediate form (SMA2). Some cases may present in adulthood, which are usually dominantly inherited. Pathologically there is loss of lower motor neurons from the spinal cord and brain stem, and remaining ones may be swollen with accumulations of neurofilaments. In SMA1 skeletal muscle shows severe atrophy, but in other forms muscle may show chronic myopathic changes, in addition to features of chronic denervation.

12.6   Hereditary Spastic Paraparesis

This is a group of inherited disorders characterised by slowly progressive spastic paraparesis associated with degeneration of the corticospinal tracts and posterior column tracts. A growing number of different genetic mutations have been described and inheritance may be dominant, recessive or X-linked and in some cases there may be additional neurological involvement.

References

1. Lambert JC, Heath S, Even G, Campion D, Sleegers K, Hiltunen M, et al. Genome-wide association study identifies variants at CLU and CR1 associated with Alzheimer's disease. Nat Genet. 2009;41(10):1094–9.
2. Bu G. Apolipoprotein E, and its receptors in Alzheimer's disease: pathways, pathogenesis and therapy. Nat Rev Neurosci. 2009;10(5):333–44.
3. Braak H, Braak E. Neuropathological stageing of Alzheimer-related changes. Acta Neuropathol. 1991;82(4):239–59.
4. Hyman BT, Phelps CH, Beach TG, Bigio EH, Cairns NJ, Carrillo MC, et al. National Institute on Aging-Alzheimer's Association guidelines for the neuropathologic assessment of Alzheimer's disease. Alzheimers Dement. 2012;8(1):1–13.
5. Gearing M, Mirra SS, Hedreen JC, Sumi SM, Hansen LA, Heyman A. The Consortium to Establish a Registry for Alzheimer's Disease (CERAD). Part X. Neuropathology confirmation of the clinical diagnosis of Alzheimer's disease. Neurology. 1995;45(3 Pt 1):461–6.
6. Savva GM, Wharton SB, Ince PG, Forster G, Matthews FE, Brayne C, et al. Age, neuropathology, and dementia. N Engl J Med. 2009;360(22):2302–9.
7. Collinge J. Molecular neurology of prion disease. J Neurol Neurosurg Psychiatry. 2005;76(7): 906–19.
8. Jackson GS, Burk-Rafel J, Edgeworth JA, Sicilia A, Abdilahi S, Korteweg J, et al. Population screening for variant Creutzfeldt-Jakob disease using a novel blood test: diagnostic accuracy and feasibility study. JAMA Neurol. 2014;71(4):421–8.
9. Gill ON, Spencer Y, Richard-Loendt A, Kelly C, Dabaghian R, Boyes L, et al. Prevalent abnormal prion protein in human appendixes after bovine spongiform encephalopathy epizootic: large scale survey. BMJ. 2013;347:f5675.
10. Parchi P, Strammiello R, Notari S, Giese A, Langeveld JP, Ladogana A, et al. Incidence and spectrum of sporadic Creutzfeldt-Jakob disease variants with mixed phenotype and co-occurrence of PrPSc types: an updated classification. Acta Neuropathol. 2009;118(5):659–71.
11. Hilton D, Stephens M, Kirk L, Edwards P, Potter R, Zajicek J, et al. Accumulation of alpha-synuclein in the bowel of patients in the pre-clinical phase of Parkinson's disease. Acta Neuropathol. 2014;127(2):235–41.

Chapter 13
Trauma

Abstract Injury to the brain and spinal cord remains the commonest cause of death in young adults in many regions of the world. This chapter describes the pathology of head and spinal cord injury, including the types of haemorrhage, diffuse axonal injury and effects of internal herniations. The pathological findings in inflicted head injury in children and chronic traumatic encephalopathy are also described.

Keywords Trauma • Head injury • Contusions • DAI

Injury to the brain and spinal cord remains an important cause of long term disability, and in Europe and North America, is the commonest cause of death in individuals under the age of 45 years. The majority of cases result from falls, road traffic accidents, assaults and contact sports. The incidence is highest in children, young adults and the elderly, and is about twice as common in males compared with females. Alcohol ingestion is often a factor in the aetiology of adult head injury.

A simple clinical assessment of the severity of head injury in adults can be undertaken using the Glasgow coma score [1]. A score of less than 9 is classified as severe head injury and is associated with a poorer outcome.

Injury to the head can be broadly classified as either missile or non-missile, with differing patterns of pathology. Non-missile, or blunt, head injury is most often caused by rapid acceleration or deceleration of the head with or without impact, and occasionally by crushing of the head. By contrast missile injuries are due to impact of the head by rapidly moving external objects such as a bullet, and may result in penetration into the cranial cavity. Blunt head injury causes both localised and diffuse brain injury, some of which develops at the time of the head injury, however secondary processes may also develop over several hours to days such as brain ischemia, hypoxia, swelling and infection. In a significant minority of patients with severe head injury, and individuals with repetitive low impact head injury, the development of chronic traumatic encephalopathy with progressive neurological deterioration years later may occur.

The outcome of head injury is related both to the severity and the nature of the initial event and patient factors such as age, co-morbidity including other injuries,

D.A. Hilton, A.G. Shivane, *Neuropathology Simplified: A Guide for Clinicians and Neuroscientists*, DOI 10.1007/978-3-319-14605-8_13

sepsis and treatment. Genetic factors also play a role and, in particular, polymorphisms for the *apolipoprotein E gene* affect the pathological changes and clinical outcome from head injury, with individuals possessing two copies of the *ε4 allele* having a worse outcome than those without this allele [2, 3].

13.1   Focal Injury

13.1.1   Scalp Injury

Lacerations, abrasions and bruising to the scalp are common and are a good indicator of the site of impact. In some cases scalp injury may give an indication of the type of object that came into contact with the head. Generally scalp lacerations are not of great clinical significance, however, they can result in profuse haemorrhage and are a potential source of infection. It should be noted that bruising is not always a result of direct impact for example periorbital bruising ('Raccoon eyes') is commonly associated with orbital roof fracturing as a result of a contrecoup injury e.g. after falling backwards and hitting the occiput, and mastoid bruising (Battle's sign) occurs secondary to fracture of the petrous temporal bone and tracking of blood, often a few days after the injury.

13.1.2   Skull Fractures

These indicate that significant force was involved in the injury, and may occur either as a coup injury being initiated at the point of impact, or as a contrecoup type injury. Contrecoup fractures commonly involving the roofs of the orbits following a fall backwards, landing on the back of the head resulting in a shockwave passing through the skull and shattering the relatively thin orbital bones. Linear skull fractures are common and radiate from the point of impact along lines of least resistance, and may involve both the calvarium and skull base. A deep linear fracture extending from side to side across the middle cranial fossa through the petrous ridges and pituitary fossa may result in a 'hinge fracture' and indicates severe side to side impact of the skull, and is usually associated with fatal head injury. A 'ring fracture' through the posterior middle fossa and encircling the foramen magnum indicates either severe hyperextension of the neck or a fall from a height, landing on the feet forcing the spinal column upwards. If a forceful heavy impact is spread over a wider surface area, the skull may be fractured into multiple fragments ('comminuted fracture'), and if over a small area, may result in a 'depressed fracture' whereby a portion of bone is pushed inwards indenting the brain which requires surgical decompression. Fractures may follow suture lines ('diastatic fracture'), particularly in childhood before the sutures are fully ossified.

Skull fractures are associated with an increased risk of intracranial infection, particularly 'compound fractures' where the overlying skin is lacerated, and also with an increased risk of intracranial haemorrhage. Fractures, particularly basal skull, may result in CSF leakage and the formation of aeroceles within the cranial cavity.

13.1.3 Brain Contusions and Lacerations

Superficial areas of bruising to the brain ('contusion'), often associated with tearing of the pia ('laceration'), are common after non-missile head injuries. Brain contusions (Fig. 13.1) usually follow a stereotypical pattern which is independent of the site of injury, with involvement of the crests of gyri, particularly involving the frontal poles, orbital surfaces of the frontal lobes, temporal poles, lateral and inferior surfaces of the temporal lobes and occipital poles. They occur commonly after rapid deceleration of the head (e.g. after falling backwards and hitting the back of the head), and are due to the continued movement of the relatively soft brain across the hard irregular surface of the skull. Contusions are less common in infants where the floor of the skull has a smooth outline. Contusions may also occur adjacent to a fracture ('fracture contusion'), or in relation to brain herniation ('herniation contusion'), such as compression of the brain against the free edge of the tentorium cerebelli or externally against the skull edge at the site of the craniectomy defect. If the area of brain contusion extends through a laceration into the subdural space then this is known as a 'burst lobe' and is most common in the frontal and temporal lobes. Bleeding into an area of contusion may continue for many hours after the initial injury, contributing to raised intracranial pressure. After a period of weeks or

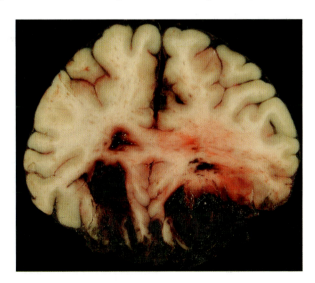

Fig. 13.1 Acute contusions, showing areas of superficial haemorrhage in the inferior frontal lobes

months the contusions will resorb, resulting in scarring and yellow/brown discolouration from blood breakdown products. Many contusions are asymptomatic, although they may be a trigger for chronic epilepsy.

13.2   Traumatic Intracranial Haemorrhage

13.2.1   Extradural Haemorrhage

This commonly occurs as a result of tearing of the middle meningeal artery in association with a fracture of the squamous temporal bone as a direct result of impact. Although the bleeding is arterial, due to the dense adherence of the dura to the inner aspect of the skull, it may take several hours for significant accumulation of blood, resulting in an initial lucid interval. Extradural haemorrhage is seen in approximately 10 % of individuals with severe head injury and is not always associated with a skull fracture, particularly in children due to the greater flexibility of the skull. The accumulation of blood is classically biconvex on imaging and requires urgent surgical drainage.

13.2.2   Subdural Haemorrhage

This results from tearing of the bridging veins crossing the subdural space, particularly those adjacent to the superior sagittal sinus. This is due to rapid deceleration of the head and continued movement of the brain within the cranial cavity stretching these short veins. It is particularly common in the elderly where brain atrophy allows greater movement of the brain within the cranial cavity. Acute subdural haemorrhage presents shortly after head injury (Fig. 13.2), however, if bleeding is slow it may present in a subacute form (1–2 weeks after injury) or as a chronic subdural haemorrhage (more

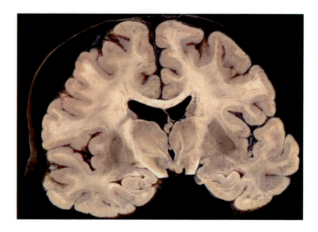

Fig. 13.2 Subdural haemorrhage overlying left hemisphere compressing adjacent brain

than 2 weeks after injury). The head injury may not be severe, particularly in the elderly, patients on anticoagulation and alcoholics. In the acute phase, haemorrhage has a 'blackcurrant jelly' appearance and after a period of several days separates into serous fluid with an organising membrane of granulation tissue on both the dural and pial surfaces, developing over 1–2 weeks. Re-bleeding may occur, possibly due to haemorrhage from newly formed blood vessels within the granulation tissue and fibrinolysis.

13.2.3 Subarachnoid Haemorrhage

Subarachnoid bleeding is commonly seen in association with contusions and lacerations. Other causes of traumatic subarachnoid haemorrhage include leakage of intraventricular haemorrhage through the exit foramen of the IV ventricle, and tearing of basal vessels in association with skull fractures. Massive subarachnoid haemorrhage may occur due to laceration of basal vessels following assault, resulting in collapse and rapid death due to tearing or dissection of basal vessels. Scarring from subarachnoid haemorrhage may result in chronic obstruction to CSF drainage and the development of hydrocephalus in long term survivors.

13.2.4 Parenchymal Haemorrhage

Superficial haemorrhage into the cerebral and cerebellar hemispheres usually is associated with contusions. However, haemorrhage in the basal ganglia, thalamus and parasagittal white matter may be seen in high impact head injuries in association with diffuse axonal injury.

13.2.5 Intraventricular Haemorrhage

Intraventricular haemorrhage usually results from extension of deep parenchymal haemorrhage into the ventricular system.

13.3 Other Localised Injury

13.3.1 Focal Vascular Injury

Hyperextension of the neck may result in vertebral or carotid artery dissection (Fig. 13.3) and carotid cavernous sinus fistula may develop resulting in pulsating exopthalmus.

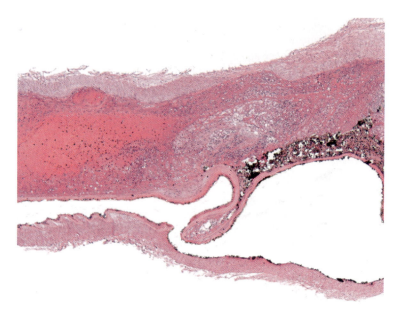

Fig. 13.3 Longitudinal section of internal carotid arteries showing traumatic dissection with haemorrhage between the media and adventitia of the upper arterial wall. H&E stain

13.3.2   Pituitary Gland Infarction

Traumatic transection of the pituitary stalk and markedly raised intracranial pressure may cause pituitary infarction.

13.3.3   Brain Stem Avulsion

Severe hyperextension of the neck may result in partial or complete avulsion of the brain stem, which usually results in immediate death. This most commonly occurs at the pontomedullary junction, but may also occur at the craniocervical junction.

13.3.4   Cranial Nerve Avulsion

Anosmia is common after head injury as a result of injury to the olfactory fibres and bulb, but damage to the other cranial nerves may also occur, including the optic, facial and auditory nerves.

13.4   Diffuse Brain Injury

13.4.1   Diffuse Axonal Injury

Traumatic diffuse axonal injury is widespread axonal damage that occurs as a result of rapid acceleration or deceleration of the head, and this is more likely when the head movement is rotational or side-to-side, rather than backwards or forwards. It should be noted that diffuse axonal injury may also occur as the result of other types of brain injury including hypoxia, ischaemia, hypoglycaemia, drugs of abuse and toxins, however, the histological patterns are somewhat different to that seen after trauma. Traumatic axonal injury most often results from road traffic accidents, but may occur from other types of injury including falls from a height and assault. If severe, traumatic axonal injury typically results in the patient being unconscious from the point of impact with a poor outcome and may result in death, disability and persistent vegetative state. Damage to the axons is often associated with small tears of capillaries resulting in petechial haemorrhages (Fig. 13.4a) and may be graded in terms of severity (Table 13.1).

Axonal damage results from stretching of nerve fibres in long white matter tracts resulting in tears in the axolemma, associated with influx of calcium triggering activation of calcium dependent enzymes causing damage to cytoskeletal proteins and axonal transport. This results in accumulation of proteins in axons, such as β amyloid precursor protein (βAPP), which may be visualised as axonal swellings after several hours (Fig. 13.4b), and eventually axotomy, with 'axon retraction balls'. Severely affected areas include the corpus callosum, parasagittal and subcortical fibres, internal capsule, cerebellar white matter and brainstem. After a period of several weeks to months there is atrophy and grey discolouration of white matter, which may be associated with cavitation and hydrocephalus *ex vacuo* (Fig. 13.5).

13.4.2   Diffuse Vascular Injury

Widespread small petechial haemorrhages are seen in the white matter of the cerebral hemispheres and brainstem in some patients who die almost immediately after head injury. The haemorrhages are due to traction of small cerebral blood vessels and survival is not long enough for the development of axonal changes.

13.4.3   Brain Swelling and Ischaemia

Brain swelling, with resulting raised intracranial pressure and reduced cerebral perfusion pressure causing cerebral ischaemia, is a common secondary complication of head injury. Brain swelling may be particularly prominent in children

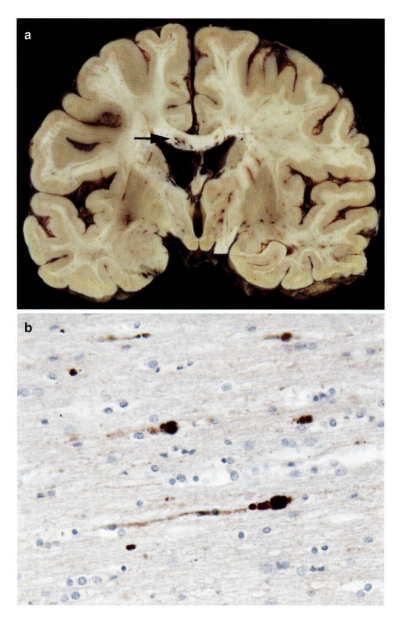

Fig. 13.4 (**a**) Acute diffuse axonal injury showing petechial haemorrhages in corpus callosum (*arrow*) (Reproduced with permission from Whitfield et al. [4]). (**b**) Accumulation of beta amyloid precursor protein in swollen axons known as 'axon retraction balls'. Immunohistochemistry for βAPP

Table 13.1 Grading of traumatic axonal injury [5]

Grade 1	Axonal damage (microscopic)
Grade 2	Axonal damage associated with haemorrhagic lesions in the corpus callosum
Grade 3	Axonal damage associated with haemorrhagic lesions in the corpus callosum and brainstem

Fig. 13.5 Chronic survivor
of diffuse axonal injury in
persistent vegetative state
showing marked loss of white
matter with grey
discolouration, cystic change
and hydrocephalus *ex vacuo*
(Reproduced with permission
from Whitfield et al. [4])

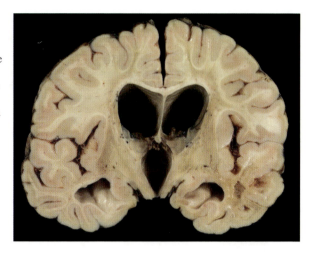

and adolescence, and in addition to the primary injury, other factors may contribute to its development including seizures, hypoxia, ischaemia and sepsis.
Any additional intracranial space occupying lesions such as haematomas, will
also contribute to raised intracranial pressure. Not all areas of the brain are
equally susceptible to ischaemia and areas of particular vulnerability include the
watershed areas between the different arterial territories, particularly the anterior and middle cerebral arteries, and in the Sommer's sector of the hippocampal
formation. In addition, brain swelling may result in internal herniation of the
brain and subsequent arterial compression: anterior cerebral artery compression
may result from subfalcine herniation of cingulate gyrus; posterior cerebral
artery ischaemia may result from medial temporal lobe and midbrain compression of the artery against the free edge of the tentorium cerebelli; brainstem
ischaemia may result from transforaminal herniation of the brainstem ('coning')
which is usually fatal.

13.4.4   Fat Embolism

Fat embolism may be seen in patients with long bone fractures with or without
head injury. It is due to the release of bone marrow emboli, which include lipids,
and occlude vessels in the lung and brain. Neurological symptoms usually
develop 2–3 days after the fracture and symptoms include dyspnoea, hypoxia and
confusion. The brain shows multiple small areas of petechial haemorrhage in the
white matter and lipid emboli can be seen within intracranial blood vessels
(Fig. 13.6).

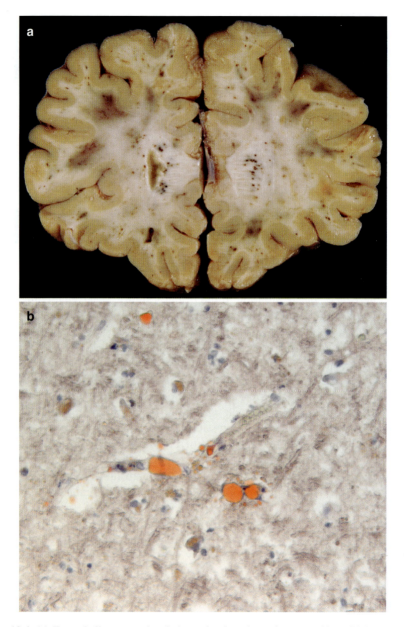

Fig. 13.6 (**a**) Fat embolism occurring 2 days after long bone fracture with multiple petechial haemorrhages within the frontal white matter. (**b**) Lipid emboli (*orange coloured*) within capillary lumen. Lipid stain

13.5   Missile Head Injury

A rapidly moving object impacting the head will usually result in focal brain injury, unless it is a high velocity missile (e.g. rifle bullet) in which case the injury may be more widespread. Missile injury may result in a depressed fracture or full penetration of the object into the cranial cavity, with focal brain damage and a high risk of infection and post traumatic epilepsy. Perforating injuries result from the object (usually a bullet) passing through the skull, and usually also through the brain. If the object is of low velocity it may ricochet within the cranial cavity and implant fragments of bone and scalp into the brain. High velocity bullets produce a shock wave causing extensive brain damage and usually a large exit wound.

13.6   Inflicted Head Injury in Childhood

Non-accidental injury to young children and infants ('shaken baby syndrome') is important to recognise. Warning signs include retinal haemorrhages (otherwise uncommon in infants more than 1 month old), retinal tears, detachments, vitreous haemorrhage, retinal folds and other unexplained injuries to a young child or infant. Characteristic pathological findings, in addition to the ocular changes, are a thin layer of subdural haemorrhage, subarachnoid haemorrhage, brain swelling, haemorrhage into the optic nerve sheaths, cervical roots and muscles of the neck. There may be evidence of traumatic axonal injury, particularly in the corticospinal tracts of the lower medulla and upper spinal cord. The relatively large head and weak neck of the infants predispose them to brain injury from shaking, even without impact, however, there is controversy about the exact mechanisms involved.

13.7   Chronic Traumatic Encephalopathy

Approximately 15 % of patients who survive severe head injury undergo progressive neurological decline decades later, and this is more common in individuals with repetitive brain injury such as sportsmen involved in contact sports (e.g. boxing, ice hockey, American football) and domestic abuse victims [6, 7]. Patients often have parkinsonian features, apathy and dementia. Pathologically, there is Alzheimer-type pathology involving the cortex and substantia nigra [6]. Interestingly, neurofibrillary tangles have been described in boxers as young as 23 years old. Fenestration of the septum pellucidum is also a common finding.

13.8 Spinal Cord Injury

Spinal cord trauma is a significant cause of disability and may result from either direct damage to the cord such as compression, contusion, laceration and haemorrhage, or secondary to hypoxia and ischaemia. Cord injury is often associated with spinal fracturing, and some patients may develop syringomyelia and meningeal fibrosis, which may result in progressive neurological decline.

References

1. Teasdale G, Maas A, Lecky F, Manley G, Stocchetti N, Murray G. The Glasgow Coma Scale at 40 years: standing the test of time. Lancet Neurol. 2014;13(8):844–54.
2. Smith C, Graham DI, Murray LS, Stewart J, Nicoll JA. Association of APOE e4 and cerebrovascular pathology in traumatic brain injury. J Neurol Neurosurg Psychiatry. 2006;77(3):363–6.
3. Sorbi S, Nacmias B, Piacentini S, Repice A, Latorraca S, Forleo P, et al. ApoE as a prognostic factor for post-traumatic coma. Nat Med. 1995;1(9):852.
4. Whitfield PC, Thomas EO, Summers F, Whyte M, Hutchinson PJ. Head injury – a multidisciplinary approach. Cambridge, UK: Cambridge University Press; 2009. p. 16. 978–0521697620.
5. Adams JH, Doyle D, Ford I, Gennarelli TA, Graham DI, McLellan DR. Diffuse axonal injury in head injury: definition, diagnosis and grading. Histopathology. 1989;15(1):49–59.
6. DeKosky ST, Blennow K, Ikonomovic MD, Gandy S. Acute and chronic traumatic encephalopathies: pathogenesis and biomarkers. Nat Rev Neurol. 2013;9(4):192–200.
7. Lehman EJ. Epidemiology of neurodegeneration in American-style professional football players. Alzheimers Res Ther. 2013;5(4):34.

Chapter 14
Paediatric Diseases

Abstract This chapter discusses the common congenital malformations and diseases occurring in the perinatal period. Paediatric neuropathology is a highly sub-specialised field of neuropathology and a good knowledge of the normal developmental processes and the ability to distinguish normal from abnormal for a particular age is essential for accurate interpretation of gross and microscopic findings. The way the developing nervous system responds to an injury varies during different stages of development. One clinical importance of recognising these conditions (especially malformations) lies in guiding genetic counselling for family members.

Keywords Malformations • Development • Perinatal • Hydrocephalus • Defects

14.1 Congenital Malformations

The CNS malformations contribute to approximately 8–10 % of still births and 5–6 % of early neonatal deaths according to one USA and Europe-wide study [1] and are a significant cause of morbidity. The severity of various malformations form a clinical spectrum with some conditions incompatible with life (e.g. anencephaly) and others causing subtle structural abnormalities resulting in epilepsy, mental retardation, learning and behavioural difficulties (e.g. lissencephaly, microcephaly, cortical dysplasia). Genetic and environmental factors have been found to play a role in the aetiology of CNS malformations.

Before discussing the common congenital malformations, a brief overview of the normal CNS development is presented and outlined in Table 14.1. The nervous system begins to develop with the formation of a neural tube from the midline ectoderm (begins around 16th post ovulation day, and is completed by 4 weeks). This process is termed *'neurulation'*. The neural tube then undergoes segmentation and cleavage to form the major subdivisions of the CNS (which is completed by 8 weeks). The last step is proliferation and migration of cells which eventually populate the various CNS regions (this occurs between 8 weeks and birth; some processes continue even after birth).

© Springer International Publishing Switzerland 2015   219
D.A. Hilton, A.G. Shivane, *Neuropathology Simplified: A Guide for Clinicians
and Neuroscientists*, DOI 10.1007/978-3-319-14605-8_14

Table 14.1 Stages of nervous system development and associated defects

\n\nNeural tube	***Neurulation*** (formation of neural tube; 16th post ovulation day until 4 weeks gestation)	*(Neural tube defects)*
		Anencephaly
		Encephalocoele
		Meningomyelocoele
		Meningocoele
		Spina bifida occulta
	Segmentation and Cleavage- (formation of major subdivisions of CNS; complete by 8 weeks)	Holoprosencephaly
		Arhinencephaly
		Agenesis of corpus callosum
		Anomalies of septum pellucidum
	Proliferation and Migration-(8 weeks- birth or later)	Microcephaly
		Megalencephaly
		Lissencephaly
		Polymicrogyria
		Neuronal heterotopia
		Cortical dysplasia

14.1.1   Neural Tube Defects

Defects of neural tube closure- Craniorachischisis is the most severe form where there is defective closure of much of the neural tube exposing the brain and spinal cord to amniotic fluid, followed by their degeneration and necrosis. *Anencephaly* results from failure of closure of anterior neuropore. The brain and calvarium are absent and is replaced by a mass of glial and vascularised tissue termed *'area cerebrovasculosa'*. Anencephalics may be alive at birth but invariably die in the new born period. The defect can be detected by ultrasound or MRI scan and is associated with raised alpha-fetoprotein in maternal serum. The incidence is high in Ireland, Wales [2], and India (Punjab), but low in Japan. Folate supplementation in women of child-bearing age has been found to reduce the risk of anencephaly [3]. Other associated abnormalities include hypoplasia of the pituitary, adrenal glands and lungs. *Myelomeningocoele* shows herniation of spinal cord and meninges through a large vertebral defect and is common at the lumbo-sacral level. Defects above T12 level are more common in females and are associated with other anomalies. Grossly, they can present as flat or cystic mass covered by skin. The histology shows intact or ulcerated, atrophic epidermis with underlying vascularised meningeal tissue containing islands of glial tissue.

Table 14.2 Chiari malformations

Chiari Type 1	Chiari Type 2	Chiari Type 3
Herniation of cerebellar tonsils through foramen magnum.	Herniation of cerebellar vermis, malformed and downwardly displaced brainstem (Fig. 14.1).	Cerebello-encephalocoele through a bony defect.
Associated with syringomyelia, skeletal anomalies such as occipital dysplasia and craniosynostosis.	Associated with lumbosacral myelomeningocoele and hydrocephalus.	Associated with brainstem deformities and lumbar spina bifida.

Axial defects with herniation of neural tube- Encephalocoele is herniation of brain tissue through a cranial defect, which occurs most frequently in the occipital region. Other less common sites include fronto-ethmoidal and parietal regions. Occipital encephalocoeles may be associated with Meckel-Gruber syndrome; a lethal autosomal recessive condition linked to chromosome 11 and 17, and also has polycystic kidneys, hepatic fibrosis and bile duct proliferation. Protrusion of only the cranial or spinal meninges through a bony defect is termed a *Meningocoele.* In a spinal meningocoele, both dura and arachnoid herniate; the spinal cord may show hydromyelia, splitting or tethering.

Tail bud defects- Spina bifida occulta is the mildest form of neural tube defect, always a closed defect, which is characterised by minor spinal cord abnormalities such as *hydromyelia* (over distension of the central canal*), diastematomyelia/diplomyelia* (longitudinal splitting or duplication of the cord) and *tethered cord.* These are most common in the lumbo-sacral region.

14.1.2   Chiari Malformations

Chiari malformations are of three types (Table 14.2) and are characterised by cerebellar abnormalities with or without hydrocephalus. The malformation may become symptomatic during infancy, teenage years or in adults. Some of the clinical features include neck or arm pain, sleep-apnoea, stridor, feeding difficulties, nystagmus, lower cranial nerve palsies, weakness and quadriparesis.

14.1.3   Disorders of Forebrain Induction

After complete closure of the neural tube, its anterior end undergoes segmentation into three vesicles- prosencephalon (which gives rise to forebrain), mesencephalon (midbrain) and rhombencephalon (hindbrain). The forebrain and hindbrain undergo further divisions into telencephalon (cerebrum), diencephalon (basal ganglia and thalamus) and metencephalon (pons and cerebellum), myelencephalon (medulla)

Fig. 14.1 Chiari type 2
malformation showing
herniation of cerebellar
vermis (*arrow*) and elongated
brainstem

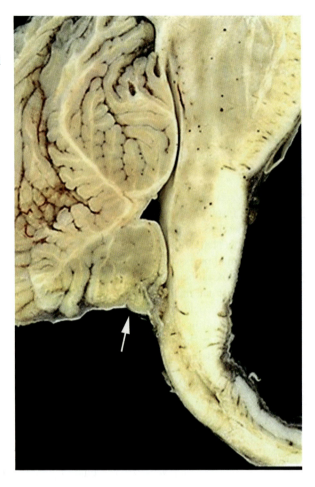

respectively. Subsequent cleavage of the prosencephalon gives rise to two cerebral hemispheres and ventricles. Several genes such as *Shh* (sonic hedgehog), *Bmp7* (bone morphogenetic protein 7) and *Emx1* play important roles in forebrain development [4–6].

Holoprosencephaly (single ventricle and single cerebrum) results from failure or incomplete cleavage of the prosencephalon. This can be sporadic or associated with trisomy's 13, 18 and triploidy. Severely affected children often die in the neonatal period. In those who survive, clinical symptoms include mental retardation, seizures, anosmia and pituitary insufficiency. Based on the severity of the malformation the following different forms are recognised: Arhinencephaly (mildest), lobar, semi lobar and alobar holoprosencephaly (severe form). In arhinencephaly, the olfactory bulbs, tracts and gyri recti are absent on both sides. In lobar form, the cerebral hemispheres are separated by inter hemispheric groove, but the cingulate cortex is continuous along the midline. The corpus callosum and olfactory bulbs are still absent or hypoplastic. The semi lobar form (Fig. 14.2) shows partially formed

Fig. 14.2 Semi lobar holoprosencephaly showing absence of corpus callosum, dilated lateral ventricle, fused thalami and absent third ventricle

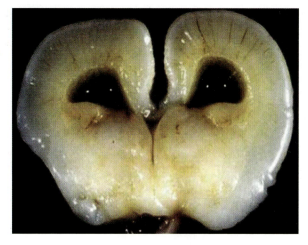

shallow inter hemispheric fissure, mainly in the posterior occipital regions. Anteriorly, there is continuity of the cingulate cortex across the midline and olfactory bulbs are usually absent. The alobar form is severest form associated with various facial anomalies. This is characterised by a globular undivided cerebrum with monoventricle, fused basal ganglia and thalami, and no olfactory structures or corpus callosum. Histology may reveal abnormalities in cortical cytoarchitecture such as polymicrogyria and neuronal heterotopias.

Agenesis of corpus callosum can be total or partial (posterior portion, splenium, absent). It can be sporadic or familial and associated with other malformations such as holoprosencephaly. The cingulate gyrus is also deficient. The corpus callosum is replaced by an abnormal longitudinal bundle (called the *'Probst bundle'*) and the angles of the lateral ventricles are upturned (*'bat wing'* appearance) (Fig. 14.3a, b).

Anomalies of septum pellucidum include *agenesis* (in association with septo-optic dysplasia- optic hypoplasia, septal aplasia and hypopituitarism), *cavum septi pellucidi* (cavity at the anterior end; incidental finding at autopsy) and *cavum vergae* (cavity at the posterior end).

14.1.4 Neuronal Migration Disorders

Lissencephaly refers to macroscopic finding of smooth brain with no convolutions (Fig. 14.4a, b), also termed *'Agyria'*. *'Pachygyria'* refers to coarse or widened convolutions. These are defects in neuronal migration and can be sporadic or familial. They are of two types- Lissencephaly I (smooth cortex) and Lissencephaly II (cobblestone cortex). Miller-Deiker syndrome is associated with type I and has mutated *LIS1* gene. Type II is associated with various cerebro-ocular dysplasias (Walker-Warburg syndrome, Muscle-Eye-Brain disease and congenital muscular dystrophy). Various genes are involved in these conditions and include- *LIS1, DCX*

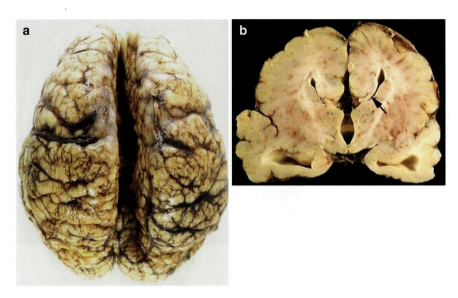

Fig. 14.3 Brain showing separated cerebral hemispheres and absent corpus callosum (*a*), coronal slice showing upturned angles of lateral ventricles and abnormal longitudinal *'Probst'* bundle (*arrow*) (**b**)

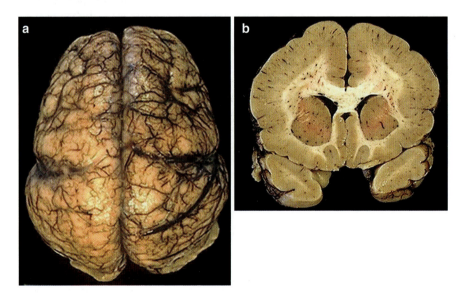

Fig. 14.4 (**a, b**) Brain showing Lissencephaly (smooth surface) resulting in absence of cortical gyri (Agyria)

(*doublecortin*), *TUBA1A, ARX, RELN, POMT1*. The genes listed above, upon their mutation, can have distinct phenotypes. The general appearance on histology is that of a four-layered cerebral cortex (instead of a normal six-layered cortex) with

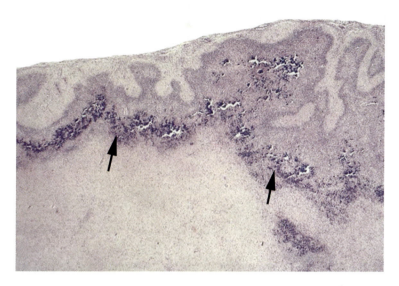

Fig. 14.5 A case of polymicrogyria showing extensive calcification (*arrows*). H&E stain

associated heterotopias in some cases. Islands of ectopic neurons are present in the subarachnoid space giving a cobblestone appearance in Lissencephaly type II.

Polymicrogyria refers to excessive folding and irregular fusion of adjacent gyri giving an abnormal appearance to cortical ribbon (*'Moroccan leather'*). They can be focal or widespread; peri sylvian region being one of the common sites. These lesions may be asymptomatic or present with severe neurologic disability depending upon their extent. They can be acquired (in association with infections and metabolic diseases) or familial (Aicardi syndrome). Its pathogenesis is presumed to be hypoxic-ischaemic and the estimate of its timing is third to fourth gestational month. Histology shows unlayered (commonest), 2-layered or a 4-layered (rare) cortex (Fig. 14.5).

Neuronal heterotopias are focal collections of neurons within the white matter. They can be diffuse, nodular or band-like (laminar heterotopia). It should be noted that it is common to find occasional neurons within the anterior temporal lobe white matter in otherwise normal brain. *Diffuse heterotopias* can be sometimes seen in epileptic patients. *Nodular heterotopias* (Fig. 14.6) are commonly seen in the periventricular regions. They can be incidental findings or associated with other malformations such as microcephaly or megalencephaly. They arise from faulty neuronal migration and an X-linked form linked to *filamin-1* gene has been described. *Laminar or band heterotopia* (or double cortex) usually occurs in females and cause mild epilepsy. It forms a spectrum with Lissencephaly type I and involves *LIS1* and *DCX* genes. The band of heterotopic grey matter lies parallel to the overlying normal cortex and separated from it by a thin strip of white matter.

Focal cortical dysplasias are abnormalities in cortical lamination and organisation and are commonly encountered in surgical resections carried out for intractable

Fig. 14.6 Coronal slice of the brain showing nodular heterotopia (*arrow*) in the left hemispheric white matter. There is also left hemiatrophy

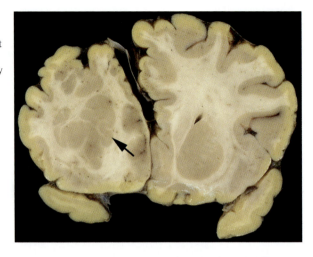

Fig. 14.7 A large porencephalic cyst over the superolateral aspect of cerebral hemisphere

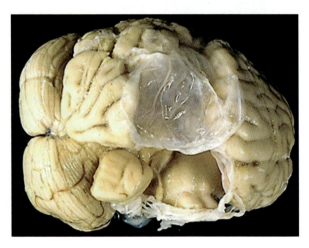

epilepsy. Recently, the International League Against Epilepsy (ILAE) classified focal cortical dysplasia into three histological types (discussed further in Chap. 8).

14.1.5   Encephaloclastic Defects

Porencephaly (Fig. 14.7) is a smooth-walled defect in the cortical mantle, commonly seen over the Sylvian fissure or central sulcus, extending from the brain surface into the ventricles. The gyri around the defect may show abnormal radiating pattern or polymicrogyria. This result from an hypoxic-ischaemic injury sustained during mid-gestation, after neuronal migration but before the development of mature cortex (i.e. after 20–24 weeks). *Basket brain* is intermediate in severity between porencephaly and hydranencephaly and shows symmetric bilateral cystic

Fig. 14.8 A case of hemi-megalencephaly showing asymmetric enlargement of left cerebral hemisphere

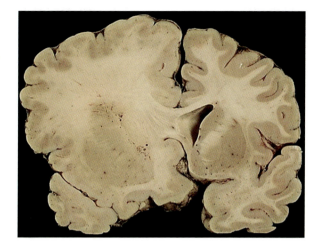

destruction of lateral frontal and parietal lobes with preserved medial cingulate cortex. *Hydranencephaly* (bubble brain) is the severest form showing cystic destruction of the entire supero-lateral cerebral hemispheres. The inferior surfaces of frontal, temporal and occipital lobes are usually spared. Hydranencephaly has been reported in association with familial Fowler syndrome (proliferative vasculopathy). Hypoxic-ischaemic insult during late gestation to early infancy results in a condition termed *'multicystic encephalopathy'* characterised by multiple cystic destructive process with associated gliosis within the grey and white matter in all lobes.

14.1.6   Microcephaly, Megalencephaly, Hemi-megalencephaly

Microcephaly (small head), used synonymously with *microencephaly* (small brain), refers to brains weighing less than 2 SD below mean, and can be an isolated finding or associated with some chromosomal disorders (Down's syndrome, fragile X syndrome), metabolic diseases (phenylketonuria), maternal infections and irradiation. *Megalencephaly* is defined as brain weights 2.5 SD above mean. Males are affected twice as often as females. They may be an isolated finding, familial or associated with various conditions (achondroplasia, sphingolipidoses, mucopolysaccharidoses, leukodystrophies, and neurocutaneous syndromes). *Hemi-megalencephaly* (Fig. 14.8) refers to asymmetric enlargement of one cerebral hemisphere. This is commonly seen in the setting of tuberous sclerosis. The various morphological abnormalities include polymicrogyria, pachygyria and focal cortical dysplasias.

14.1.7   Cerebellar, Brainstem and Spinal Cord Malformations

Table 14.3 lists the various hindbrain and spinal cord malformations-

Table 14.3 Hindbrain and spinal cord malformations

Cerebellum	Brainstem	Spinal cord
Agenesis or hypoplasia	Olivary heterotopia	Syringomyelia (Fig. 14.9a, b) or syringobulbia
Dandy-Walker syndrome (agenesis of vermis, dilated 4th ventricle, enlarged posterior fossa and hydrocephalus)	Olivary and dentate dysplasia	Abnormal decussation of pyramidal tracts
Chiari malformations	Mobius syndrome (aplasia or hypoplasia of cranial nerve nuclei, calcification, peripheral neuropathy, myopathy)	Arthrogryposis multiplex congenita (foetal hypokinesia resulting in multiple contractures)
Joubert syndrome (agenesis of vermis, occipital meningocoele)		
Pontoneocerebellar hypoplasia		
Granule cell aplasia		
Heterotopias and cortical dysplasias		

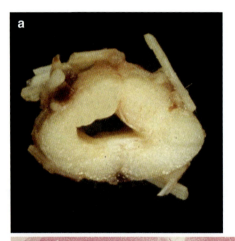

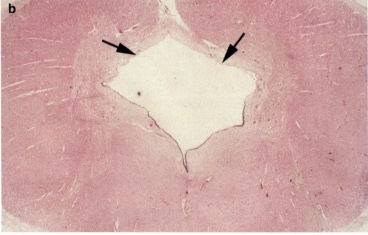

Fig. 14.9 Syringomyelia showing dilated central canal (**a**), and focal absence of ependyma lining the central canal (*arrows*) (**b**). H&E stain

14.2   Hydrocephalus

Hydrocephalus refers to increase in the volume of CSF within the cranial cavity. This can occur due to increase in CSF production, reduced absorption or by blockage of CSF flow or drainage. Some of the common causes of hydrocephalus in children are listed in Table 14.4.

Aqueductal stenosis (characterised by a very tiny lumen) or *atresia* (with many tiny canals or aqueductules) (Fig. 14.10) and *aqueductal gliosis* can result in CSF flow obstruction and hydrocephalus. Stenosis can be sporadic, X-linked or rarely autosomal recessive. The X-linked form shows characteristic absence of medullary pyramids. Atresia may be sporadic or associated with other anomalies like Arnold-Chiari malformation, hydranencephaly, craniosynostosis or infections. Both stenosis and atresia show absence of gliosis in the surrounding tissue. *Choroid plexus papilloma* can cause hydrocephalus by CSF oversecretion or by obstructing CSF flow. Intrauterine and neonatal infections (such as Toxoplasmosis, Gram-negative bacteria, fungi), intraventricular haemorrhage and mucopolysaccharidoses can cause fibrotic occlusion of CSF pathway resulting in hydrocephalus.

14.3   Perinatal Diseases

14.3.1   Hypoxic-Ischaemic Neuronal Injury

Neuronal damage resulting from hypoxia and/or ischaemia is the most common pathological process seen in paediatric post-mortems. The severity of the injury depends on several factors such as regional blood flow, selective vulnerability of neurons, nature, duration and timing of insult. The various aetiological factors for hypoxic/ischaemic lesions include: maternal diseases (abruption, cardiac arrest, anaemia), drugs, smoking, trauma, placental and cord abnormalities (haemorrhage, infarction, infection, short or long cord), and congenital diseases (heart, lung, metabolic, malformations). The neuronal injury can be widespread affecting all cerebral regions or may show specific patterns which are exclusive to the perinatal period (pontosubicular necrosis, thalamus-brain stem injury, *status marmoratus*/basal ganglia). The

Table 14.4 Causes of hydrocephalus in children	Obstruction of aqueduct of Sylvius
	Choroid plexus papilloma, other extrinsic/intrinsic neoplasms
	Absence of arachnoid granulations, Ciliary dysplasia
	Dandy-Walker and Chiari malformations
	Arachnoid cysts
	Infection, Haemorrhage and post-inflammatory scarring
	Ventriculomegaly (associated with Holoprosencephaly, Hemimegalencephaly, Lissencephaly)
	Hypoxic-ischaemic and degenerative lesions (grey or white matter)

Fig. 14.10 Aqueduct atresia with many tiny canals or aqueductules. H&E stain

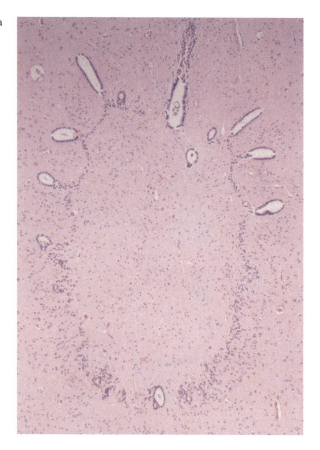

morphological changes associated with hypoxia and/or ischaemia is different in the developing immature brain compared to a mature adult brain. The hypoxic changes in the developing brain manifest as nuclear fragmentation (karyorrhexis), and not as cytoplasmic eosinophilia (red neurons) (see Chap. 2) seen in adults. In chronic lesions, the dead neurons may become encrusted with calcium or iron (ferrugination).

14.3.2   White Matter Lesions

Periventricular leukomalacia (PVL) is commonly seen in premature infants and is pathologically characterised by focal periventricular necrosis, associated reactive gliosis and microglial activation. The white matter injury most likely results from ischaemia-reperfusion or cytokine release during ischaemia or infection. The imma-ture oligodendroglial precursors are selectively vulnerable in the perinatal period and therefore result in impaired myelination. The end stage is a solid glial scar or a cavity with reduced white matter volume. The PVL lesions may co-exist with other lesions of hypoxia-ischaemia such as neuronal necrosis or haemorrhage. The incidence of cystic PVL has reduced with the introduction of modern neonatal intensive care and is now considered to be an uncommon finding on brain imaging. The cause for this shift from cystic to non-cystic PVL is not known. The long term effects of PVL include hypomyelination and clinical motor deficits of cerebral palsy.

14.3.3   Cerebral Haemorrhages

The periventricular germinal matrix and the ventricles are the most common sites for intracerebral haemorrhage in a low birth weight premature infant. The germinal matrix is a thick layer of closely packed progenitor cells which give rise to immature neurons and glial cells. It also contains thin walled blood vessels which are vulnerable to rupture and haemorrhage. The haemorrhage can be recognised with cranial ultrasound and the severity can be graded. A venous origin has been identified for most haemorrhages [7]. The blood in the ventricles then spreads to the subarachnoid space, causes hydrocephalus and elicits an inflammatory reaction. The end result is destruction of germinal matrix with cyst formation. As the germinal matrix harbours important progenitor cells, their destruction leads to various cytoarchitectural abnormalities in the surrounding brain tissue.

The other less common sites of intracerebral haemorrhage in the perinatal period include choroid plexus and cerebellum. Other causes for intracerebral haemorrhage include- trauma, coagulation abnormalities, vascular malformations, and haemorrhage within a tumour.

14.3.4   Hypoglycaemia

Neonatal hypoglycaemia is likely to have serious adverse effects on brain growth and other organs. The incidence is higher in premature, than full-term, births. Infants at risk for hypoglycaemia are those with reduced glycogen stores (e.g. premature infants, stress, asphyxia, glycogen storage disease), hyperinsulinism (e.g. diabetic mothers, pancreatic tumours, exchange transfusion, drugs) and reduced glucose production. The occipital lobes and insula are found to be preferentially affected. The neuropathological changes observed appear to be diffuse and widespread affecting neurons as well as glial cells. The classic ischaemic neuronal changes (red neurons; see Chap. 2) noted in adult hypoglycaemic brain damage is rarely seen in the neonates. The microscopic changes in neonates include nuclear shrinkage, pyknosis, karyorrhexis, chromatolysis and cytoplasmic vacuolation.

14.3.5   Kernicterus

Kernicterus means 'yellow discolouration' of specific grey nuclei within the brain of infants suffering from severe jaundice. This is due to accumulation of unconjugated/free bilirubin. Bilirubin which forms from the breakdown of blood is normally conjugated by the liver, secreted in bile, deconjugated in the intestines and excreted in faeces. Immaturity of the conjugating enzymes in the neonates and various other predisposing conditions lead to increased levels of free bilirubin, which readily crosses the blood-brain barrier and causes neurotoxicity. The brain in patients dying from kernicterus shows symmetrical bright-yellow discolouration in different regions which include- globus pallidus, thalamus, subthalamus, hippocampus, cranial nerve nuclei, substantia nigra, locus coeruleus, dentate nuclei, Purkinje cells and spinal cord. Early lesions show neuronal and neuropil vacuolation, eosinophilic change and chromatolysis. Later stages show neuronal loss, gliosis and macrophage infiltration. Kernicterus can be treated or prevented by reducing hyperbilirubinaemia.

14.3.6   Infections

CNS infections common in the perinatal period include bacterial meningitis (Group B *Streptococci, E. coli, L. monocytogenes,* Gram-negative bacteria, *H. influenzae,* Meningococcus, Pneumococcus), fungal infections (Candidiasis and occasionally *Mucor, Cryptococcus, Coccidioides, Aspergillus*) and TORCH (*T*oxoplasmosis, *O*thers. e.g. syphilis, *R*ubella, *C*ytomegalovirus, *H*erpes simplex or *H*IV) group of infections. (Refer to Chap. 5 for details on these infections). The outcome of these various infections on the human brain depends on the timing of infection; teratogenic effects are seen in infections during early gestation when the brain is still developing, whereas more destructive inflammatory process is seen in infection acquired at later stages of gestation or in newborn period when the brain has developed enough to respond to the infection.

14.3.7   Rare Neurodegenerative Diseases

Neurodegenerative diseases presenting in childhood are rare and mainly affect the grey matter. These include Alpers-Huttenlocher syndrome (affects cerebral cortex and liver), Familial striatal degeneration (affects basal ganglia), Neurodegeneration with brain iron accumulation type 1 (previously termed Hallervorden-Spatz disease', see Chap. 12), Menke's disease, Ataxia-telangiectasia, Carbohydrate-deficient glycoprotein syndrome type 1 (CDG 1), Cerebellar degenerations, Infantile neuroaxonal dystrophy, Leigh's disease (see Chap. 11), and Spinal muscular atrophy (see Chap. 9).

References

1. Kalter H. Five-decade international trends in the relation of perinatal mortality and congenital malformations: stillbirth and neonatal death compared. Int J Epidemiol. 1991;20(1):173–9.
2. Nevin NC, Johnston WP, Merrett JD. Influence of social class on the risk of recurrence of anencephalus and spina bifida. Dev Med Child Neurol. 1981;23(2):155–9.
3. De-Regil LM, Fernandez-Gaxiola AC, Dowswell T, Pena-Rosas JP. Effects and safety of periconceptional folate supplementation for preventing birth defects. Cochrane Database Syst Rev. 2010(10):CD007950.
4. Rubenstein JL, Beachy PA. Patterning of the embryonic forebrain. Curr Opin Neurobiol. 1998;8(1):18–26.
5. Dale JK, Vesque C, Lints TJ, Sampath TK, Furley A, Dodd J, et al. Cooperation of BMP7 and SHH in the induction of forebrain ventral midline cells by prechordal mesoderm. Cell. 1997;90(2):257–69.
6. Hayhurst M, McConnell SK. Mouse models of holoprosencephaly. Curr Opin Neurol. 2003;16(2):135–41.
7. Ghazi-Birry HS, Brown WR, Moody DM, Challa VR, Block SM, Reboussin DM. Human germinal matrix: venous origin of hemorrhage and vascular characteristics. AJNR Am J Neuroradiol. 1997;18(2):219–29.

Chapter 15
Autopsies

Abstract Autopsy continues to have an important role in allowing a better understanding of the causes of death and underlying diagnosis in many patients with neurological diseases. In the context of neurosurgery, autopsy is a valuable means of audit of death, and many neurodegenerative diseases cannot be diagnosed with accuracy during life. It is important that legal and ethical criteria are followed when undertaking autopsies.

Keywords Autopsy • Consent • Audit

Autopsy continues to have a significant role in allowing a better understanding of a patient's illness and the relevant factors that led to an individual's death and remains a valuable tool in the audit of patient care [1, 2]. Before an autopsy can be undertaken it is important that appropriate legal and ethical conditions have been met, and these vary between countries. In many jurisdictions an autopsy may be requested under the authority of a Coroner or police in the case of a suspicious, work-related or 'unnatural' deaths, where there may be legal proceedings or financial compensation involved. However, if a death is regarded as due to a natural disease, a 'consented' autopsy may be undertaken. For ethical, and in many countries, legal reasons, permission from the relative's next-of-kin should be obtained prior to undertaking autopsy examination (unless consent had been given during life by the deceased). During the consenting process the family should be informed of the benefits of undertaking the autopsy and, in general terms, what an autopsy involves, which may include retention of organs such as the brain, spinal cord and various tissue samples. The requirements for tissue and organ retention vary from case to case and prior discussion with the pathologist is advised. Where whole brain retention is undertaken, examination is best undertaken after the brain has been fixed in formalin so that it is firm enough for relatively thin sectioning. Brain fixation usually takes between 2 and 6 weeks, depending on the method used, which will result in a delay to the issuing of reports.

A request for autopsy should be made to the pathology department which should include full clinical history, the particular questions that the clinical team would like answered from the autopsy, and any potential for hazard group 3 pathogens

© Springer International Publishing Switzerland 2015   235
D.A. Hilton, A.G. Shivane, *Neuropathology Simplified: A Guide for Clinicians and Neuroscientists*, DOI 10.1007/978-3-319-14605-8_15

(e.g. HIV, hepatitis B or C, tuberculosis, CJD), which will require the pathologist and mortuary staff to take additional precautions. Patients with suspected group 4 pathogens should only have autopsies in highly specialised units.

In the case of neurosurgical deaths an autopsy can be very helpful in understanding what led to the patient's death, particularly in post-operative/peri-operative deaths, and in the case of tumours allow for a more accurate assessment of the extent of the tumour within the nervous system and elsewhere in the body. The results of these autopsies should be discussed at mortality meetings with clinical teams, so that the information derived from them can be used to improve the quality of future patient care. In many neurological disorders autopsy still is the primary means of providing a definitive diagnosis (e.g. most neurodegenerative disorders [3]), but also in many other types of disease, including stroke [4]. A definitive diagnosis may be helpful to the clinical team and better understanding of the patient's response (or lack of) to any treatment provided, and an understanding of their neurological presentation. Many neurodegenerative disorders are familial and an accurate diagnosis provides families with useful information, and in a growing number of cases, will allow genetic testing of frozen brain tissue. Autopsy allows the examination of many tissues and therefore the assessment of the extent of systemic involvement of primary CNS disorders, for instance autopsy study has confirmed the peripheral involvement in Parkinson's disease and variant CJD. Autopsy also provides a range of tissues which cannot be obtained during life, which may be used for research that leads to a better understanding of neurological disorders.

Many neurological disorders now have dedicated brain banks whereby disease and control tissue are collected primarily for research. Brain banking of large numbers of cases of particular disorders has facilitated an improved understanding of disease pathogenesis and a classification, and for instance has led to the much more detailed classification and better understanding of the frontotemporal dementias.

Autopsy examination may also be helpful in muscle and nerve disorders. In the case of muscle disease it allows a assessment of the extent of muscle involvement, as sampling may be taken from multiple muscle groups and cardiac and smooth muscle and also involvement of other systems such as the central nervous system. Many histochemical techniques work well on autopsy muscle tissue, even if it is undertaken several days after death. Peripheral nerve is not generally well preserved post mortem and assessment of demyelinating conditions in particular may be difficult. However, it may provide useful information particularly in relation to inflammatory nerve disease, vasculitis and amyloid. It also allows assessment of both central and peripheral nervous system involvement.

References

1. Moorchung N, Singh V, Mishra A, Patrikar S, Kakkar S, Dutta V. Is necropsy obsolete – an audit of the clinical autopsy over six decades: a study from Indian sub continent. Indian J Pathol Microbiol. 2013;56(4):372–7.

2. Roulson J, Benbow EW, Hasleton PS. Discrepancies between clinical and autopsy diagnosis and the value of post mortem histology; a meta-analysis and review. Histopathology. 2005;47(6):551–9.
3. Love S. Neuropathological investigation of dementia: a guide for neurologists. J Neurol Neurosurg Psychiatry. 2005;76 Suppl 5:v8–14.
4. Love S. Autopsy approach to stroke. Histopathology. 2011;58(3):333–51.

Appendix 1. Suggested Reading

1. Dickson DW, Weller RO. Neurodegeneration- the molecular pathology of dementia and movement disorders. 2nd ed. ISN, Hoboken: Wiley-Blackwell; 2011.
2. Dubowitz V, Sewry CA, Oldfors A. Muscle biopsy- a practical approach. 4th ed. Saunders: Elsevier; 2013.
3. Ellison DW, Love S, Chimelli L, Harding BN, Lowe JS, Vinters HV, Brandner S, Yong WH. Neuropathology- a reference text of CNS pathology. 3rd ed. Elsevier: Mosby; 2013.
4. Goebel HH, Sewry CA, Weller RO. Muscle disease- pathology and genetics. 2nd ed. ISN, Chichester, West Sussex: Wiley-Blackwell; 2013.
5. Louis DN, Ohgaki H, Wiestler OD, Cavenee WK. WHO classification of tumours of the central nervous system. 4th ed. IARC: Lyon; 2007.
6. Love S, Perry A, Ironside J, Budka H. Greenfield's neuropathology. 9th ed. vol. 1 & 2. CRC Press, London; 2015.
7. Vallat JM, Weiss J. Peripheral nerve disorders- pathology and genetics. ISN, Chichester, West Sussex: Wiley-Blackwell; 2014.

© Springer International Publishing Switzerland 2015   239
D.A. Hilton, A.G. Shivane, *Neuropathology Simplified: A Guide for Clinicians and Neuroscientists*, DOI 10.1007/978-3-319-14605-8

Index

© Springer International Publishing Switzerland 2015
D.A. Hilton, A.G. Shivane, *Neuropathology Simplified: A Guide for Clinicians
and Neuroscientists*, DOI 10.1007/978-3-319-14605-8

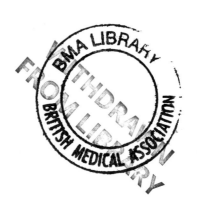